SEX, LIES AND PHARMACEUTICALS

RAY MOYNIHAN

& DR. BARBARA MINTZES

SEX, LIES
+
PHARMACEUTICALS

HOW DRUG COMPANIES PLAN TO PROFIT FROM FEMALE SEXUAL DYSFUNCTION

GREYSTONE BOOKS

D&M PUBLISHERS INC.

Vancouver/Toronto/Berkeley

First published by Allen & Unwin Pty Ltd,
83 Alexander Street, Crows Nest, Sydney, NSW, 2065, Australia

10 11 12 13 14   5 4 3 2 1

Greystone Books
An imprint of D&M Publishers Inc.
2323 Quebec Street, Suite 201
Vancouver BC Canada V5T 4S7
www.greystonebooks.com

Cataloguing data available from Library and Archives Canada
ISBN 978-1-55365-508-4 (pbk.)
ISBN 978-1-55365-652-4 (ebook)

Cover design by Jessica Sullivan
Cover photograph © Ashley Jouhar/cultura/Corbis
Printed and bound in Canada by Friesens
Text printed on acid-free, 100% post-consumer paper
Distributed in the U.S. by Publishers Group West

We gratefully acknowledge the financial support of the Canada Council
for the Arts, the British Columbia Arts Council, the Province of British
Columbia through the Book Publishing Tax Credit, and the Government of
Canada through the Canada Book Fund for our publishing activities.

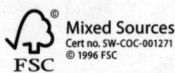

Mixed Sources
Cert no. SW-COC-001271
© 1996 FSC
FSC

*For Toni, who is body surfing the waves of time with
her turtle, adorned with the emu feathers falling from the stars . . .
in celebration of your fearlessness and strength, your warmth
and generosity, your laughter and love.*

CONTENTS

Author's note

Sex seems to be how most of us got here, apart from the odd case of an immaculate conception or a miracle of medical technology. Sex is also something that—just like the weather—most of us are interested in, more or less. But just so you're under no illusions, while this book is certainly about sex, it's also an exposé of how medical science is imperceptibly merging with pharmaceutical marketing.

As a disclosure front and centre, for more than a decade I've been writing about the tangled web of relationships between doctors and drug companies, and the unhealthy impacts of that entanglement on people and public health systems. My co-authored 2005 book describing that problem, *Selling Sickness: How drug companies are turning us all into patients*, laid out ten case studies of disease-mongering: the process of widening the boundaries of illness in order to sell people more treatments. With humility and surprise, I can report that *Selling Sickness* has since been translated into twelve languages, and reprinted a number of times in North America and elsewhere.

In *Sex, Lies and Pharmaceuticals* the making of a single modern medical condition is forensically examined, and the resulting story is both fascinating and frightening. The book's methods are those of rigorous investigative journalism, targeted at uncovering what happens behind the scenes of contemporary medical science. It draws on many scientific journal articles, medical textbooks, historic works of philosophy and sexuality, as well as some juicy corporate marketing materials and a few very revealing court documents.

I have also interviewed a long list of the key players in the emerging field called 'sexual medicine', spoken to professors, psychologists, bloggers, doctors and drug company insiders, and attended scientific seminars and medical meetings all over the world. The facts and evidence have been checked meticulously, and an extensive notes section has been included at the end of the book. I should apologise in advance to those who may feel there's too much detail at certain points, but for others this will be the lifeblood of the story. And if you do find a factual error, please let us know so we can correct it in future editions.

Almost everyone approached for an interview agreed to speak with me, and their comments have been invaluable, with many appearing in direct quotations. While a tiny handful declined—as is noted when necessary—every effort has been made to fairly represent their viewpoints, which are readily available through their many publications and presentations.

It is important to say very clearly here that the book does not accuse anyone of lying. The 'lies' in the title refers to the fictions that flow from pharmaceutical marketing—like the notion that one in ten women suffers from a disorder of low desire. As we'll see, soon that disorder itself may no longer even exist. The corporate need to market drugs for discrete disease labels does not match well with uncertainty over how to understand and classify women's sexual difficulties.

One practical note for the reader is that the terms 'dysfunction', 'disorder' and 'disease' are used regularly, sometimes interchangeably, as these are the words employed by drug companies and some doctors to describe many of the sexual problems women experience. Others involved in the debate about sex tend to use another set of words, like 'difficulties', 'dissatisfactions' or 'discontent', instead of the more medical language. Trying to define the difference between a difficulty and a dysfunction is an extremely challenging task and, as uncovered in the following pages, one that is generating a compelling global debate.

Most importantly, the book readily acknowledges that women's sexual problems can sometimes be disabling, and proven therapies—including pills—may be extremely valuable for some people. Yet it also asks very directly how much discontent is being manufactured through the creation of new sexual norms, and how much dissatisfaction is being exploited for corporate gain.

Finally, *Sex, Lies and Pharmaceuticals* is offered by co-author Barbara Mintzes and me as an opportunity to join this global debate about the making of a new medical condition. It is part of a conversation, its ideas to be discussed with family and friends, criticised in book clubs and on blogs and debated at public meetings around the world. Please join in, and feel free to bring tomatoes, a copy of the book for signing, or both.

Ray Moynihan
Byron Bay, June 2010
www.raymoynihan.net

Sex, lies and pharmaceuticals

Not tonight, dear, the dog ate my testosterone patch.

—*Dr Leonore Tiefer*

During the last year or so, has there been a period of several months or more when you lacked interest in having sex? When you felt anxious about your sexual performance or were unable to achieve an orgasm? Was there an extended time when you had trouble getting aroused, experienced pain on intercourse or just didn't find sex pleasurable? If you answered 'yes' to just one of these survey questions, and you're a woman, you could easily be classified as suffering from a brand new medical condition called 'female sexual dysfunction', or FSD. First described in the textbooks only a few decades back, FSD is set to become the next blockbuster medical condition, coming soon to a doctor's surgery near you. As the ups and downs of daily life are re-categorised as the symptoms of medical diseases, soon all of us will be sick.

One of the women who actually helped write the definitions of female sexual dysfunction puts it very clearly. '[W]hat once was considered normal,' wrote American psychologist Sandra Leiblum, 'has come to be considered dysfunctional.'[1] Nowadays, if a woman lacks the desire for sex, and is bothered by it, she could be diagnosed with a disorder of low libido. That's just one of the four main disorders of female sexual dysfunction described in one of the leading manuals of diseases.[2] The others include disorders of arousal, orgasm and pain. As the evidence plainly shows, forces are fast amassing to tell you, and your doctor, that close to one in every two women suffers from some form of this new medical condition.

The giant pharmaceutical industry—with worldwide sales now approaching a trillion dollars a year—is hungrier than ever for new markets.[3] In order to maximise sales, the industry must 'create the need' for its newest and most expensive products. Sometimes that means selling sickness to the wealthy healthy, helping transform common ailments into widespread conditions that require treatment with the latest pills.[4] Applauded for producing medicines that extend life and ameliorate suffering, drug companies no longer simply sell drugs; they increasingly sell the diseases that go with them.

Female sexual dysfunction is perhaps the perfect example of selling sickness, and the commercial firepower behind its forthcoming promotion is simply awe-inspiring. 'With more than 50 million potential sufferers in the United States, FSD could offer a larger market than male sexual dysfunction,' wrote a pair of enthusiastic market observers. 'FSD could be the next boon for pharma companies . . .'[5] If a drug is approved to treat this condition in the United States, the tsunami of marketing that will be unleashed in the media and on the web will soon swamp the shores of nations everywhere. According to industry reports, one company on the verge of having its product approved for women had set aside $100 million for the drug's advertising budget alone.[6]

Three global corporations in particular have been at the forefront of the race to spread the word about this new medical condition, and get their drugs approved to treat it. Pfizer, the biggest pharmaceutical company in the world and currently worth well in excess of $100 billion, has had high hopes that its wonder drug for men, Viagra, will also work for women. Procter & Gamble, with global annual sales of almost $80 billion, is famous for selling soap to housewives, but it also wanted to sell them testosterone patches as well.[7] The third corporation featuring in this drama is the family-owned German outfit Boehringer, which boasts just over forty thousand employees and has affiliated companies in almost 50 countries. The German company's pill targets the brain, with claims it can give women back their lost desire.

So what exactly is this condition called FSD? The answer depends a little on the solutions being sold at the time you ask the question. If Pfizer is promoting a drug that enhances blood flow to the genitals, then the condition might best be described as an 'insufficiency' of vaginal engorgement. If Procter & Gamble is pushing its testosterone patch as a cure for women, the sexual disorder is discussed as a 'deficiency' of hormones. And if Boehringer has a pill that affects the mind's neurotransmitters, women with low libido may have a 'chemical imbalance' in their brains. In a strange way, the disease seems designed to fit the drug.

That's not to say that medicines don't have a role to play in treating some sexual problems. There are women for whom a medical label and a medication may be extremely valuable. The problem is that when the drug company-sponsored tsunami of marketing reaches its full fury in your corner of the planet, women's common sexual difficulties will likely be portrayed not as aspects of normal sexuality, but as the symptoms of medical conditions that are widespread and treatable with pills. The fact that sexual difficulties are often caused by a raft of complex factors, from relationship stresses to religious taboos, may well be washed away in the coming flood of pharma-funded magazine features, celebrity interviews on breakfast TV and plain-talking advice from sexy bloggers. The first unmistakeable signs of this marketing are already appearing. 'What is female sexual dysfunction?' asks one online personality known as Katie, on her educational website. 'This health problem is a genuine problem that needs medical attention. Most women suffer from this problem without actually realising it.'[8]

Yet even before the king tide of corporate marketing has really begun to flow, a backlash has been brewing. Working out of her small home office in Manhattan, not too far from the headquarters of the world's biggest drug giant, a smart feminist scholar has launched a pre-emptive strike. Together with a small group of colleagues, sex therapist and New York University associate professor Dr Leonore Tiefer has started a grass-roots campaign. The fight is against what Dr Tiefer and her colleagues see as Big Pharma's attempt to help turn the ordinary ups and downs of women's sex lives into medical diseases in order to sell them drugs. Instead of a medical dysfunction with four neat sub-disorders, the campaigners are proposing a radically different approach to understanding women's sexual difficulties.

As we'll learn, during the extended combat there have been many colourful skirmishes, like the time Leonore Tiefer won a major award from her peers in the sex research community and delivered a speech titled 'Not Tonight, Dear, the Dog Ate My Testosterone Patch'.

Pushed for a public response to the criticisms, the powerful pharmaceutical industry has been uncharacteristically shy, rejecting the idea that it creates diseases and arguing simply that it is sponsoring a legitimate field of medical science. For their part, the doctors and psychologists who work closely with the industry believe they're raising awareness of the under-recognised suffering of women with a genuine sexual dysfunction. More importantly, they say, they're helping to give those women access to much-needed treatments.

The broader context for this extraordinary fight over female sexuality has been the paradox, in Western countries at least, of an increasing sexual openness accompanied by what appears to be a growing sexual anxiety. The promise of sexual emancipation in the heyday of the 1960s has been followed in subsequent decades by a rising tide of sexual uncertainty. *Sex and the City*'s Samantha may well climax more often than many of the female characters who came before her, but she lives in a world where pornography has moved from being a subterranean undercurrent to front and centre in the mainstream of advertising and culture. Males may, on the whole, be more sensitive now than they were in the 1950s, but post-Viagra they're bombarded by marketing messages telling them real men must be eternally ready for action. Confident female media stars provide powerful new models for teenage girls, yet the unhealthy sexualisation of girl children has become a major scandal. Young women might be winning more often in the classroom, but in the bedroom many are expected to remove their pubic hair as a prerequisite for successful sexual activity. And with the popular Brazilian waxing exposing all, cosmetic surgeons are promoting a nip and tuck to tidy up the labia, while online companies offer a genital colorant that 'restores the pink back to a woman's genitals'.[9]

When they land, the seeds of the corporate-backed campaign to transform common sexual difficulties into medical conditions will fall on the fertile ground of considerable female insecurity. Yet backward-looking moral panic about a permissive society may not be a helpful response. Perhaps it would be better to confront the reality of women's sexual dissatisfactions head on, tease out the cultural processes exacerbating their vulnerabilities, and identify the commercial forces seeking to exploit them. The dramatic story documented in *Sex, Lies and Pharmaceuticals* calls for a much greater scepticism towards simplistic claims that women's sexual difficulties are somehow due to chemical deficits rather than a complicated set of causes, including the way we relate to each other, our cultures, and our individual and collective histories. With much attention to detail, this book seeks to enable you to make your own decisions about whether to accept the labels your doctor might soon offer you, or reject them if they're not needed by viewing them as the latest products brought to you by one of the most sophisticated and profitable marketing machines on the planet.

So what exactly is all this marketing, and what form will it take? In some ways, the answer depends on where you are in the world. In the United States, drug company television advertisements will likely be the most popular way of telling people about the new disorders of sexual desire. In other places, the public face of this promotion will take a more subtle form, like an interview with an academic discussing his latest survey of sexual dysfunction. Behind the scenes, however, the drug companies are already helping to build the scientific foundations of this big new condition. As we'll discover, experts with financial ties to drug companies have been conducting sponsored surveys, designing diagnostic tools and educating your local doctor about this 'widespread' condition. And when you look closely at the small print in the disclosure sections of a plethora of medical journal articles about FSD, you'll find something even more extraordinary. Drug companies are no longer just passively funding these important milestones in the making of a new disease; in some cases, their employees are actively engaged in constructing the basic building blocks of this whole new field of medicine.

Fundamental to the building of this new science are the special relationships between the drug companies and the leading researchers. These are the respected doctors and esteemed psychologists who've actually helped revise the medical definitions of female sexual dysfunction and its four disorders. When one distinguished group of researchers sat down to refine the definitions of FSD, 95 per cent of them had financial relationships with the drug companies hoping to develop drugs for the very same condition.[10] The conflicts of interest for this group were clear. As they met to work out what could best be described as normal female sexuality, and what might better be labelled as a dysfunction, many of them had been taking money or receiving other support from companies with an interest in seeing the boundaries of this new condition broadened as widely as possible. In the end, that group chose to define FSD as arising from biological, psychological and interpersonal causes, and claimed it was 'highly prevalent', potentially affecting '20% to 50% of women'.

Once you have a workable definition of a new dysfunction, you need the surveys to confirm just how widespread it is among the general population. Commonly, that has meant asking women how often they experience things like lacking interest in sex or having trouble getting aroused. By simply ticking the box that says 'yes' in these surveys, a woman can be classified as having a condition—even though she may not even see herself as having a sexual difficulty, far less a medical dysfunction. The totals of all those little ticks in the 'yes' box are then presented as evidence of alarmingly high rates of women suffering, and scientific proof for a new epidemic. The survey findings will then be followed by the inevitable claims of a massive 'unmet need' for new treatments, including the drugs made by the company that might happen to have sponsored the survey in the first place.

The next building block to be laid into the scientific foundations of this new dysfunction is the toolkit that doctors need to measure women's pleasure and diagnose their sexual disorders. Health professionals are increasingly poking and probing women in their most intimate spaces, in the research labs and commercial clinics out on the new frontier of what's called 'sexual medicine'. With ultrasounds, doctors have been measuring the flow of blood to a woman's clitoris; with blood tests, they're assessing the levels of her testosterone; and with high-tech imaging machines, they are trying to track the reactions in her brain. At the same time, a battery of new questionnaires is being created to gauge a woman's sexual success. Yet, while the results of all these tests can appear to offer a woman objective evidence of her sexual dysfunction, there are serious questions about how useful many of the test findings really are. If a potentially dangerous drug improves your desire scores by a few points on a company-funded scale, is it really that meaningful? The facts are stark and incontestable: drug companies have started to help design the very tools used to diagnose these new disorders in your doctor's surgery. Those same tools could then provide millions of women with a medical label, opening the door to widespread prescribing of the sponsor's drug.

Next comes the 'education', during which your family physician learns about the latest definitions, the survey findings and the new diagnostic tools at company-sponsored seminars featuring company-sponsored speakers. From universities in the American Midwest to prestigious international meetings in Paris, drug company money is providing the platform for much of what our health professionals see and hear about women's sexual problems. In a fundamental way, corporations driven solely to maximise their drug sales are helping to shape the science of the new sexual disorders, even before their drugs are approved to treat them. The company executives are not actually writing the technical definitions of female sexual dysfunction, but they are bankrolling its creation as a looming twenty-first-century epidemic. This merging of marketing and medical science is not a conspiracy; it's all entirely legal. And for the time being at least, it's also perfectly acceptable under the self-regulatory codes of conduct governing the behaviour of scientists, doctors and drug companies. Many might think it's unhealthy, but with pharmaceutical companies still funding medical associations, patient advocacy groups and even universities, change may be some time coming.

This emerging field of sexual medicine is, after all, no different from almost every other corner of the medical establishment, which—as many of us are already aware—is entangled in a vast web of financial relationships with the drug or device makers. It is important to remember, though, that just because a doctor works as a consultant or speaker for a company doesn't mean he or she becomes a paid stooge for the sponsor, or conducts lesser quality science. This is not a case of individual professionals somehow changing what they say or do because they're being paid for specific pieces of work by industry. Usually doctors and drug companies choose to collaborate as partners because of their shared enthusiasm for finding new treatments. The relationships are mutually beneficial, with the companies in need of the doctors' expertise and credibility as much as the doctors are in need of the industry's research funding or consultancy fees.

Still, as a result of all these collaborations, in the broad church of differing scientific opinions, people with particular perspectives are provided with influential platforms. Certain voices are amplified through company press releases and medical journal articles, via prominent presentations at scientific conferences and educational seminars, and through the hundreds of millions that may soon be spent on drug company advertisements for new medicines. The cumulative effect, according to the people who study these relationships, may well be a systemic pro-drug bias in contemporary medical science and a gross distortion in the wider public debate about sex.

The other obvious problem is that the patient is too often left out of this picture. Too often the worlds of our leading medical experts are lubricated with drug company largesse, the friendly marketing staff constantly picking up the tab for the doctor's food, wine, travel and accommodation. Far too frequently, the scientific debates about how to understand and treat sexual problems are taking place in restaurants or lecture halls sponsored by those with a financial interest in widening the reach of a condition, and narrowing the range of solutions offered to treat it.

Apart from sponsoring many of the surveys, questionnaires, seminars and conferences, the drug companies have also been doing a lot of old-fashioned drug testing. They've been trialling different sorts of medicines to try and fix women's sexual problems: trying to get more blood flowing to the genitals, boosting testosterone levels or correcting those so-called chemical imbalances in the brain. A slow trawl through the medical literature reveals the industry has been busy funding many studies, including full-scale placebo-controlled trials enrolling thousands of women around the world. But by and large, the much-anticipated female aphrodisiac seems to have remained an elusive fantasy.

The industry has bumped up against an unexpected enemy, surprisingly enough in the shape of one of its own pills. The humble placebo, or dummy pill, appears to be holding its own in the company-funded drug trials, causing great consternation in the corridors of medical power. It turns out that for a lot of women said to suffer with sexual dysfunction, a dummy pill may be just as good as the company's drug in helping bring modest improvements to their sex lives. The plans being hatched to finally beat that placebo once and for all are yet another fascinating thread in the story of the making of this new medical condition.

The placebo, though, is not the only problem facing those who want to portray common sexual difficulties as sexual disorders. The campaign kicked off by Leonore Tiefer and her feminist colleagues has quickly gained traction around the world, scoring high-profile media coverage of its own, running education programs for health professionals, and winning influential friends among the mainstream of the sex research community. What started as guerrilla warfare has become a full-blown battle over how we understand and deal with what is going wrong in our bedrooms.

Being sceptical about marketing messages, though, doesn't mean ignoring sexual problems that might benefit from being addressed. Pain associated with sex, for example, is common and can be extremely troubling. As many women already know all too well, seeking help for such problems—also known as dyspareunia or vaginismus—can prove extremely challenging, because in some places there is such poor understanding of the causes and potential solutions. Sadly, much of the recent high-profile scientific activity sponsored by the drug industry appears to focus more on problems of desire and arousal, with the expectation that these complaints might be more amenable to drug treatment.

In a sense *Sex, Lies and Pharmaceuticals* is less about the sex and more about the lies and pharmaceuticals: the the fictional narratives that flow from the marketing in all its visible and hidden forms. The big picture in this story will reveal how the industry is helping to manufacture new norms and market sexual disorders, trying to create a climate where drug solutions to sexual problems are frequently sought. It will offer evidence to support what others have so astutely observed: that the goal of much modern marketing is not only 'to make people dissatisfied with what they have, but also with who they are'.[11] And it will show how a small grass-roots campaign is exposing and challenging that process. It's a picture projected on to a giant global canvas, but it will also illuminate the most intimate spaces of our lives for both women and men. As we uncover the details of this captivating conflict, we can't help but reflect on our own sexual situations—the delights and uncertainty, the pleasures and pain. As Simone de Beauvoir wrote half a century ago in her feminist classic *The Second Sex*, 'in sexuality will always be materialised the tension, the anguish, the joy, the frustration, and the triumph of existence'.[12]

Sex, Lies and Pharmaceuticals makes no assumptions about the sexuality of its readers. It assumes instead the infinite variation that is the reality and the beauty of human sexuality. While most of us live with partners, many of us live alone and a significant minority of us are now single. Most of us are attracted to the opposite sex, though many of us aren't, and for others sex is simply not on the agenda. Some of us are enjoying regular love-making with a new partner, while others among us find joy in an occasional encounter during a long-term loving relationship. As a work of investigative journalism, the book offers compelling insights into the making of this particular condition. But once you identify the common patterns of disease promotion here, you'll see the strategies appearing more and more often elsewhere with other conditions, as the boundaries of treatable illness are inexorably widened. It is important to note that this book does not assume we are passive victims of that promotion or the many other powerful forces at work within our cultures. On the contrary, the detail in the pages that follow is designed deliberately to inform and empower its reader in the face of a coming corporate onslaught.

One of the benefits of drilling into all this detail about sexual disorders is that when you get up close, the very foundations of the conditions start to look decidedly shaky. Similarly, a close reading of the current medical literature reveals that tolerance of the entanglement between doctors and drug companies is waning within the ranks of the scientific establishment itself. Unease about the blurring of medicine and marketing appears to be growing steadily. High-profile reports are finding that the web of financial ties with industry can bring the risk of 'undue influence' on doctors' decisions, potentially jeopardising the care of their patients, the integrity of scientific studies and the objectivity of medical education.[13] As *Sex, Lies and Pharmaceuticals* goes to print, there are calls for a major clean-up coming from senior figures within the worlds of politics and medicine. But let's not get ahead of ourselves. Let's start the story at the point when excitement about the next billion-dollar disease was first beginning to build.

One

Difficulties or dysfunctions?

We're hoping to be able to expedite the process ... of disease
development ...

—Drug company manager Darby Stephens

The woman looking confidently into the camera lens must
be in her late twenties or early thirties, her long black hair
falling over strong shoulders, a slip of striped blue material tied
into a bow around her neck. Her red lips and good looks are
striking, but it's her words that are most captivating. Her name
is Darby Stephens, and she's a research manager at a California-
based drug company called Vivus. The company is testing a
drug for women said to suffer from a new condition called
female sexual dysfunction or FSD. As Darby Stephens explains
in an extremely candid on-camera interview for a documentary,
FSD is so new that the drug company itself has had to help
work out what the condition actually is: 'In order for us to

develop drugs, we need to better and more clearly define what the disease is,' she said.[1]

The frankness of the comments may be unusual, but the marketing activity being described is becoming commonplace. Pharmaceutical companies now assist in shaping the very diseases their drugs are targeting. Through its close ties to the medical profession and its influence over public debate, the industry is now helping to determine whether we see our sexual problems as everyday difficulties or medical dysfunctions, and whether female sex drugs become a permanent feature in the bedrooms of our future.

The Californian company where Darby Stephens was manager of clinical research had started testing a pharmaceutical cream for women to rub on their genitals, to see whether it could enhance blood flow and boost their level of sexual arousal. Before the drug testing could go into full swing, however, there was a problem that needed to be addressed. As Stephens tells it, in order to get a drug formally approved and have insurance companies pay for its use, it has to be shown to work against a specific medical condition: 'The whole thing is kind of complicated because you have to have a disease before you can treat it.'

The difficulty with FSD was that no one was really certain exactly what the condition was, and some people even questioned whether it existed at all. So part of Vivus's role, Darby Stephens explained, was to sit down with the experts, the 'thought leaders' in the field, and work with them directly on developing this new dysfunction in order to be clearer about what it was. During her frank interview, she revealed that in the 'process of defining the disease, we've been able to get thought leaders involved in female sexual dysfunction, and really work closely with them to develop this disease entity, so that it makes sense'. Her comments were made at a time when drugs for male sexual dysfunction had already been approved, and billions of dollars' worth were set to sell every year. So from the industry's perspective, there was no time to waste in developing the sister condition for women. 'We're hoping to be able to expedite the process of drug development and of disease development,' she told film-maker Liz Canner during the interview for Canner's documentary *Orgasm Inc.*

Bizarre as it may sound, the idea that a drug company would play a role in 'disease development' is backed up by observations from another industry insider, this one with expertise in the practice known as 'condition branding'.[2] The advertising expert Vince Parry famously revealed how drug companies are sometimes involved in 'fostering the creation' of medical disorders, giving a little known condition renewed attention, helping redefine or rename an old disease, or sometimes assisting in the creation of a whole new one. The branding expert has said that as part of his high-level work for drug companies he will sit down with medical experts to try to 'create new ideas about illness and conditions'. As the Canadian writer Naomi Klein told us in her classic *No Logo*, corporations are no longer just selling products, they are selling brands, and brands are about lifestyles and concepts, not commodities.[3]

These revelations about drug company plans to accelerate the development of a disease, in order to test and sell drugs for it, herald the opening of a new chapter in the story of the modern medical marketplace, where the corporate sector now works together with leading medical experts to help tell us who's sick and who's in need of the industry's latest cures. But to what extent are women's problems of desire and arousal really the signs of dysfunctions, or rather common sexual difficulties being portrayed as diseases in order to sell drugs?

One place to start answering the question is to take a closer look at the actual technical definitions of this new sexual dysfunction and its four sub-disorders. Just as some infectious diseases are technically defined by the presence of particular levels of antibodies in the blood, so too dysfunctions and disorders are defined by certain behaviours or characteristics considered abnormal. While we might imagine these medical definitions to be solid and certain, nothing could be further from the truth. This condition is poorly defined and its definitions are constantly shifting and moving—a fact readily acknowledged even by those who write them. Dr Sandra Leiblum, the high-profile psychologist from the Robert Wood Johnson Medical School with first-hand experience of revising the definitions, has eloquently described these shifting sexual sands: 'the classification of female sexual dysfunction', she wrote, 'is somewhat arbitrary, imprecise, and changeable'.[4]

One of the first things that strike you about this technical definition is that it comes from the *Diagnostic and Statistical Manual of Mental Disorders (DSM)*, which is produced by the American Psychiatric Association, the professional body representing psychiatrists. When it was first released in the 1950s the manual was a small book, but it has become a giant text running to almost 1000 pages, full of many different disorders. While it was an American creation, it is now highly influential around the world. As some readers will already know, the *DSM* is seen as something of a bible of diseases by many doctors; however, it is also regarded as controversial, coming under heavy criticism for turning the experiences of ordinary life into the signs of medical illness.[5] In its pages, severe pre-menstrual pain has become 'pre-menstrual dysphoric disorder', a set of common children's behaviours re-packaged as 'attention deficit hyperactivity disorder' and extreme shyness has been transformed into 'social anxiety disorder'. The *DSM* has also been criticised for the closeness between the expert committees who write the definitions of diseases and the pharmaceutical companies that sell the drugs prescribed to treat them. One study that looked closely at the affiliations of the men and women on those committees found that more than half of them had ties to drug companies. On the committees revising mood disorders, including depression, the figure was closer to 100 per cent.[6]

It was only as recently as the 1980s that the term 'sexual dysfunction' first appeared in the *DSM* though sexual 'disorders' had been previously listed. Since then, the definitions have changed a number of times, as the manual has been updated and new editions have been published. The details of the most recent definitions now run to many pages, but in simple terms the condition known as female sexual dysfunction, or FSD, has been divided into four sub-disorders: desire, arousal, orgasm and pain. The disorder of low desire is defined as a deficiency in sexual interest or fantasy, and technically described as 'hypoactive sexual desire disorder', or HSDD. Arousal disorder is described as inadequate genital lubrication and swelling, in response to sexual excitement. It is termed 'female sexual arousal disorder', or FSAD. 'Female orgasmic disorder' is the label attached to a woman whose orgasms are delayed, or who is unable to reach them. Pain disorder involves pain associated with sex, problems also known as dyspareunia or vaginismus. One of the criteria for each of these disorders is that women must be distressed or bothered by their situation in order to qualify for a formal diagnosis from a doctor.

Using these definitions as a foundation, different groups have revised and rewritten their own versions, as researchers struggle to find the words that accurately describe what goes wrong for women sexually. As to the causes of this 'dysfunction', the conventional medical view readily acknowledges that psychological and social factors play a big role in sexual difficulties. A woman may, for example, lose interest in sex when she's grieving the loss of a loved one, or if she's been sexually assaulted. Couples can also grow apart over time, and it may be difficult to talk about what's happening in a relationship. But the medical view is also highly interested in what are regarded as possible biological causes: problems with blood flow to the genitals, low testosterone levels or chemical imbalances in a woman's brain.

Many researchers have been content to work with the existing definitions of the four sub-disorders in the *DSM*, and to tinker with them occasionally to try to make them more accurate. Some have suggested the need for a major overhaul of the way the condition is defined.[7] Others claim FSD and its four sub-orders simply don't exist as they are defined, and the *DSM* approach to classifying women's sexual problems is fundamentally flawed.

Sex therapist and academic Dr Leonore Tiefer and other experts have argued that the definitions in the psychiatrists' manual are unhelpful because they're far too narrowly focused on problems relating to 'function'. They say the definitions fail to place a woman's sexual problems in the broader context of her life, her relationships, and the wider society and culture in which she lives. The grass-roots campaign Tiefer has helped create, called the New View, has proposed and published an alternative approach, complete with books, a website and an active global list-serve.[8]

According to the New View definition—written by a group of psychologists, academics and experts in women's health—women identify their own difficulties, which are defined as 'discontent or dissatisfaction with any emotional, physical, or relational aspect of sexual experience'.[9] Unlike the definitions in the *DSM*, this approach puts more emphasis on trying to understand the causes of a woman's sexual dissatisfaction, and on attempting to prevent them if possible. The differing approaches reflect a long-standing tension in the world of psychiatry and psychotherapy between those more interested in uncovering the root causes of problems, and those with an emphasis on describing and classifying the symptoms. In sharp contrast to the more medical view favoured by drug companies, Leonore Tiefer doesn't generally see sexual problems as individual dysfunctions that can be fixed with medications—though she and her colleagues are not opposed in principle to the idea of drugs, if safe and effective medicines emerge.

Under the New View's alternative approach, the causes of women's sexual difficulties are divided loosely into four categories. The first includes the broad factors at play in a society that impact on sexuality. These are the religious taboos that breed shame about our bodies, the cultures that help create our inhibitions and the economic factors that leave many women exhausted after combining work and family obligations. The second category of causes includes factors relating to partners, including the common mismatch in the level of desire between partners and other relationship difficulties. The third category is when sexual problems arise from psychological issues, like past abuse or depression. The fourth and final category is when sexual difficulties arise from medical causes, like nerves being damaged in surgery, or the harmful sexual side-effects of anti-depressant drugs, which can impair a person's ability to orgasm. These four categories are not mutually exclusive, and an individual woman's difficulties may well be caused by a complex interaction of more than one factor. While it rejects the idea of a widespread dysfunction, there is no sense that this approach plays down the distressing or debilitating nature of these problems for some women.

The tune the New View is singing is clearly not music to the ears of drug companies, whose pills can do little to change religious taboos or relationship woes. Portraying a sexual problem as an individual woman's failure to 'function' makes a drug solution much more appealing. A perspective that puts women's difficulties firmly in the context of their life and loves, their cultures and societies is far less valuable to those trying to promote new medicines.

The debate about what constitutes a normal part of sexual life and what should be classified as a dysfunction is not only a fascinating contemporary fight, it has a long and rich history. Dive back into the murky waters of the nineteenth century Victorian era and you'll find that homosexuality, masturbation and oral sex were all considered abnormal, deviant and diseased. Unbelievably, it was only in the 1970s that homosexuality was finally removed from the pages of the *DSM*.

By the start of the twentieth century, many Victorian-era ideas about sexual deviance and disease were under attack. Writers at that time, including Havelock Ellis, are credited with helping to usher in a more modern way of thinking about sex. Unlike influential thinkers in the nineteenth century, Ellis fought against linking everyday behaviours like masturbation to medical conditions. Seen as a champion of tolerance, Ellis was also a great enthusiast. Sex was 'the chief and central function of life', he wrote, 'ever wonderful, ever lovely'.[10] Importantly, he also challenged some of the views of his contemporary, Sigmund Freud.

One of Freud's particularly troubling theories was that women who couldn't have a 'vaginal' orgasm via intercourse were essentially childlike and immature, a gross misunderstanding of female sexuality that would cast a chill shadow over women's sense of themselves as sexual beings for much of the following century. 'The leading erotogenic zone in female children is located in the clitoris,' Freud announced in one of his essays published in 1924. 'But it appeared to me,' he wrote a year later, 'that the elimination of clitoridal sexuality is a necessary precondition for the development of femininity.'[11]

In contrast, Havelock Ellis argued that the clitoris was central to female sexuality, and he ridiculed Freud's notion that adult female sexuality was exclusively vaginal. Yet it took at least half a century before these ideas about the centrality of the clitoris became more widely accepted. For many decades of the twentieth century, women were considered to suffer from the psychiatric illness called 'frigidity' if they were not able to experience an orgasm vaginally while having intercourse.[12]

An article published in the influential *Journal of the American Medical Association* in 1950 pronounced that frigidity was 'one of the most common problems in gynaecology'. It suggested that up to 75 per cent of women derived little or no pleasure from the 'sexual act', which in most cases was because they were suffering with 'frigidity'.[13] Any condition claimed to affect up to 75 per cent of all women should raise alarm bells for us: could this really be an abnormality or malfunction if it is something that affects nearly everyone? Echoing Freud's theories, the doctors wrote that in girl children 'the clitoris gives sexual satisfaction, while in the normal adult woman the vagina is supposed to be the principal sexual organ'. According to these theories, if the normal transference of sexual satisfaction from clitoris to vagina didn't take place, then the woman had 'frigidity', the disorder defined as 'the incapacity of women to have a vaginal orgasm'. Though the term is rarely used today, it seems the ghosts of frigidity may still haunt much current misunderstanding of female sexuality.

By the mid-twentieth century, though, a fresh breeze was beginning to blow into popular sexual understanding, due in part to the famous work of Alfred Kinsey and his colleagues at Indiana University. Based on lengthy face-to-face interviews with more than 10 000 people, Kinsey and his team produced two major works on sexuality, the first book on men and the second on women, published in 1953.[14] The findings were explosive for their time, revealing that many men and women engaged in pre-marital sex, extra-marital affairs and—God forbid—homosexuality. While the term 'frigidity' was still being widely used to label women, Kinsey didn't like it at all.

> The failure of a female to be aroused or to reach orgasm during coitus [intercourse] is commonly identified in the popular and technical literature as 'sexual frigidity'. We dislike the term, for it has come to connote either an unwillingness or an incapacity to function sexually. In most circumstances neither of these implications is correct.

Rather than suffering from some supposed psychiatric disorder called frigidity, Kinsey found that most of the women he interviewed masturbated, almost all of them relied primarily on stimulation of the clitoris, and most reached orgasm that way almost all of the time. In other words, most women in his survey were both willing and able to function sexually, despite claims from within the medical profession at the time that up to 75 per cent might suffer from a sexual disorder. Their sexual dissatisfactions clearly had more to do with the way sex was happening for them, including the inadequacy of the stimulation they were receiving from their male partners, than some psychiatric condition. As to Freud's theory, still widely accepted in the 1950s, that women could transfer the site of sexual satisfaction from the clitoris to the vagina, Kinsey dismissed it as a biological impossibility.

The work of Kinsey was attacked from all sides—not only by those unable to accept the rich variety of human sexual behaviour he uncovered, but also by those accusing him of poor statistical methods and having an unrepresentative sample. Others believed he and his team put too much focus on the physical, rather than the psychological, aspects of sex. Notwithstanding the criticisms, one of the great legacies of Kinsey's work is his celebration of the wide variation in human sexuality, and his view that imposing uniform standards of what should be considered normal or abnormal performance is not only impractical but also unjust.[15]

While Kinsey's work on women was hitting bookshops across the United States, in London in 1953 an English translation of a French work of philosophy was just being published. Simone de Beauvoir's feminist text, *The Second Sex*, painted a sad, angry, despairing portrait of women still aspiring to and struggling to achieve full membership of the human race. 'The female is a female by virtue of a certain lack of qualities,' de Beauvoir quoted the Greek philosopher Aristotle as saying, 'so we should regard the female nature as afflicted with a natural defectiveness.'[16] There is a disquieting similarity between Aristotle's description of women as defective and contemporary suggestions that half of all women have a sexual dysfunction.

Simone de Beauvoir's weighty classic wasn't all doom and gloom, however. One of the book's latter chapters imagines a future inhabited by the 'independent woman'. It excitedly suggests that the 'free woman is just being born' and that she must 'shed her old skin and cut her own new clothes'. Well aware of the extent of women's dissatisfaction with their sex lives, the French philosopher was hopeful that the growing feminist activism would ultimately bring genuine equality, which might also improve sex. 'New relations of flesh and sentiment of which we have no conception will arise between the sexes,' dreamt de Beauvoir.

The French feminist's dream helped set the scene for the sexual revolution of the 1960s, in which women in many places felt freer to express themselves sexually, and the birth control pill allowed them to do so without fear of pregnancy. However, with genuine equality between the sexes still elusive, the newfound freedom to have sex also had a downside: the expectation that women were now more available for sex, whether they were interested in the idea or not. Theories about sexual difficulties were being developed against the backdrop of the tensions between a growing freedom and a continuing inequality between the sexes. Women might have had more sexual choices, but many were still in unequal relationships, often economically dependent on their male partners, and in some cases staying in abusive relationships because they couldn't see a way out.

As the 1960s rolled around, changing times and technology meant that much of the next act in the dramatic history of sex research was caught on film. Starting not long after Kinsey's explosive book on women was published, American medical researchers William Masters and Virginia Johnson began what would become their world-famous laboratory investigations. Their team would ultimately film hundreds of men and women engaged in sexual acts, including intercourse and masturbation. They would document more than 10 000 orgasms, measuring all manner of physiological responses, trying to gain insights into the nature of sex.[17] Their work produced detailed descriptions of the major changes in the human body associated with sex, like blood flow to the genitals, vaginal lubrication and nipple hardening, as well as the celebrated phenomenon of the multiple orgasm. Based on their measurements, the pair described a 'sexual response cycle' that included the four phases: excitement, plateau, orgasm and resolution. Their observations of the patterns of sexual arousal and orgasm, similar in men and women, played a key role in further developing scientific understanding of sex. They also influenced the controversial definitions of 'female sexual dysfunction' that would emerge decades later.

Masters and Johnson also did their bit to shatter myths about sex and older women. 'Nothing could be further from the truth,' they observed, 'than the oft-expressed concept that aging women do not maintain a high level of sexual orientation.'[18] While older women experience physical changes like a thinning of the skin of the vaginal walls and a slowing in lubrication, these researchers found no decline in the functioning of the clitoris, which their observations had confirmed as central to the female orgasm.[19] In other words, the changing frequency of sexual activity over a woman's life, or the slowing down that can come during a long relationship, were not necessarily the same as a decline in the capacity to function sexually.

Like Kinsey, Masters and Johnson didn't like the word 'frigidity', and they chose instead to use words considered then to be less judgemental like 'inadequacy' or 'dysfunction'. As for the sources of people's sexual problems, the couple saw a complex set of causes, including physical or biological factors. But even though they were working within a medical framework, they also emphasised the psychological, social and cultural causes of sexual problems—including forces like religions, responsible for so much guilt and shame. These cultural causes, they said, more often than not placed a woman in a position where 'she must adapt, sublimate, inhibit or even distort her natural capacity to function sexually'.[20]

These comments about women 'inhibiting' and 'adapting' their sexuality foreshadowed debates that would appear much later about how to define women's sexual troubles. Where drug companies are now trying to portray an individual with low desire as having a disorder to be fixed with pills, others see the normal behaviour of a healthy woman adapting to her surroundings, whether that might be an unhappy relationship, an early experience of abuse, or simply the pressures of trying to juggle the toddlers, the job and a chronic lack of sleep. No one dismisses the pain of a woman distressed by a debilitating lack of desire, or by the damage to her relationship that can come if her partner is saddened or angered by it. The question is how to best describe, understand and deal with it.

Delving into the debates about the causes of sexual difficulties can be both intriguing and frustrating. While one learns a lot about the reasons for dissatisfaction and discontent, it is rarely clear what the best ways to address them might be. Something receiving a lot of public attention at the moment is the decline in desire that can happen at different times during a relationship. It goes without saying that sexual interest waxes and wanes over time, depending on where you are in life, whether you're single or with a partner, and the point at which you are in a relationship. But this specific challenge of maintaining a healthy and happy sexual life within a long-term relationship has been a key interest of many sex researchers, including Alfred Kinsey. His view was that men and women in relationships tend to want a range of partners and sexual experiences, a point emphasised colourfully in the Hollywood film of his life, *Kinsey*.

'Reconciliation of the married individual's desire for a variety of sexual partners and the maintenance of a stable marriage presents a problem which has not been satisfactorily resolved in our culture,' says Liam Neeson, the actor playing Kinsey.[21] The words are uttered during a presentation given to his peers, moments before he collapses under the combined weight of the attacks being waged on his work and the sheer enormity of the task of trying to understand human sexuality. Half a century later, though the idea of lifelong marriage has faded considerably since the 1950s, the issue of the waxing and waning of desire in a loving relationship remains resolutely unresolved. Couples obviously go through periods of more or less sex, depending on whether they're relaxing on vacation or straining under the weight of work stresses. However, as Leonore Tiefer argues, the pharmaceutical industry is putting more focus on the waning of sexual interest as a problem, helping to construct the idea that a more constant and consistent level of desire is somehow the norm. 'It's sinister and it's insidious,' she says.[22]

Back when William Masters and Virginia Johnson were writing their books, Viagra, the blue pill for boys, wasn't yet even a twinkle in a marketer's eye. Back then, sex therapy was seen as one of the main solutions for sexual problems. Masters and Johnson's influential model of couple therapy, developed at their clinic in St Louis, involved both members of the couple and two therapists working intensively for a matter of weeks. Masters and Johnson claimed that this approach was very effective, though they are known more for their research and publications than for the rigour of their scientific self-assessment, so we're not really sure how well their sessions worked.

'It is to be hoped that human sexual inadequacy . . . will be rendered obsolete in the next decade,' Masters and Johnson wrote optimistically in the opening to a book they published in 1970.[23] The hope of successfully battling the species' sexual inadequacy in the space of a decade is certainly an honourable one, but it seems just a little unrealistic. It is worth reflecting, though, that these sorts of optimistic sentiments about treating, preventing and ultimately eradicating sexual problems are rarely heard any more, with corporations so reliant on selling drugs to people long term. If sexual problems were capable of being done away with via short bursts of intensive therapy, there would be no lucrative markets for the ongoing use of expensive drugs. In the 1970s, though, the pharmaceutical solutions were still some way off.

In 1976 the world's understanding of female sexuality took another step forward with the publication of *The Hite Report*.[24] Written by the feminist and educator Shere Hite, the report featured many explicit and engaging personal revelations about sexual experiences gathered from hundreds of women. Its key messages included that most woman could most easily reach climax through direct clitoral stimulation, that intercourse alone didn't generally provide enough to do the job, and that women who were unable to orgasm vaginally were in no way frigid, inadequate or dysfunctional. Like most major works on sexuality, the report has been heavily criticised, not least for its unrepresentative sample; however, its influence is unquestioned. Hite's book sold millions of copies, was translated into many languages and took pride of place on bookshelves all over the planet.

Needless to say, despite growing sexual awareness, the quaint hope that all our sexual inadequacies would be eradicated by the year 1980 didn't come to pass. The emphasis on sex therapy and the benefits of counselling as a way of dealing with sexual problems continued, but by the early 1990s a monumental change was coming to the world of sexuality. Researchers testing an experimental heart drug accidentally discovered it could increase blood flow to the genitals, and men's erections could be improved as a result. Viagra burst on to the scene and the biggest drug company in the world launched one of the most successful marketing campaigns in human history. Advertised at first by an aging politician as a treatment for a medical condition called 'erectile dysfunction', suffered predominantly by older men, the marketing of the drug was quickly transformed. In no time, television and magazine advertisements in the United States were portraying Pfizer's Viagra as a necessary sexual accessory for men of any age. As the marketing slogan told us, the pills could offer *powerful performance when you want it*.[25] A medication morphed into a sex aid, and a new multi-billion dollar market was born. So too were lively debates about the pros and cons of Viagra, credited with rekindling the love affairs of older Americans and criticised for narrowing the global conversation about sexuality to the hardness of a man's erection.

Viagra didn't just pump up penises, it also helped bring a new legitimacy to those who studied sexual problems. As the film of Kinsey's life showed, it wasn't so long ago that sex researchers were frozen out of the mainstream of science and denied funding by government health authorities. In the late 1980s, leading voices were lamenting the fact that the study of sex was still sorely missing the 'scientifically respectable apparatus' of having its own academic departments and professors of sexuality. There were calls to create a rigorous new 'sexual science', with sound methods of doing both qualitative and quantitative research using reliable measurement tools.[26] With the arrival of Viagra in the 1990s the fortunes of this field turned very rapidly around, as that 'scientifically respectable apparatus' began to be constructed. The drug industry soon extended the warm hand of friendship and funding, bringing sex researchers in from the cold and dark and helping them to build a whole new science of what's becoming known as 'sexual medicine'.[27] For doctors and psychologists working in the area, the new wonder drug was something that would not only help their patients; it might also lift up an entire field of health research.

Even before the drug was officially launched for men, plans were underway to test it in women. The problem was that, unlike men—where success could be measured by the hardness of a man's penis—it wasn't exactly clear how to measure sexual pleasure in a woman. Should it be the size of her swelling clitoris, the number of her orgasms or her feelings of sexual arousal? At that point, a decision was made to gather together a small group of researchers who specialised in women's sexuality, to start getting some answers. It would prove to be an historic gathering.

The quality of the light is one of the things that strike you first about Cape Cod in Massachusetts, in the northeast corner of the United States. It's as if you can see things more clearly from there. The wildness of the beaches, the sensuality of the sunken meadows and the clean waters of the pristine ponds are a world away from the hustle and bustle of busy Boston and metropolitan America, a couple of hours up the highway. The Cape's beauty has long attracted artists, travellers and holidaymakers, and in the spring of 1997 it brought together a very important group of doctors, sex researchers and drug company officials.

They'd been assembled with the aid of a charismatic psychologist called Ray Rosen.

A tall, handsome man, Dr Rosen is highly regarded for his intelligence and clarity of vision. Friendly and well-connected, Rosen was at the time based at the Robert Wood Johnson Medical School in New Jersey, not far from New York, Pfizer's home town. In the 1990s, while still testing Viagra, the company had been looking to make wider connections in the academic community, and Rosen would have appeared as a natural fit—particularly with his expertise in designing measurement tools, including questionnaires. Rosen would also have seen benefits in making links with a big pharmaceutical company. Apart from the funding for individual research projects and consultancies, the industry's money could help raise the profile of the whole area of sex research, ultimately helping men and women with better care. It also presented a chance to get in on the ground floor and work with this revolutionary new approach to treating sexual dysfunction. Drugs were already around that could be injected into the penis to help men's erections, but Pfizer's new blue pill worked via a different, far more convenient, mechanism. Soon the New Jersey academic entered into a working relationship with the world's biggest drug company.

As a psychologist, Ray Rosen was aware of the potential of counselling, and like many of his medical colleagues he shared what is known as a 'bio-psycho-social' approach to understanding and treating sexual problems that is both comprehensive and holistic. He was also enthusiastic about the possible role of prescription drugs for both sexes. Given what researchers knew from Masters and Johnson's observations about the similarities in male and female sexual response, and the important role of genital blood flow in both sexes, it was theoretically possible that

Viagra's benefits for men could apply equally to women. For Rosen and many of his colleagues, new opportunities for both research and treatment were opening up before their eyes, and they would grasp them with enthusiasm and energy.

Before long, it wasn't just Pfizer in the race: numerous drug companies were looking to develop their own experimental medicines, including the Californian outfit Vivus, which had high hopes its genital cream could sexually arouse millions of women. The industry was looking to make links with 'thought leaders' to help guide its drug development and raise awareness of FSD. Like health professionals across all areas of medicine, Ray Rosen embraced the chance to collaborate with industry— as would many others. The sort of the collaboration he had in mind was spelled out very clearly in an email he sent to one of his colleagues around this time, his old friend Leonore Tiefer.

Warm, gregarious and highly eloquent, Tiefer was already something of an identity in this small field, and both she and Rosen had already served terms as office holders of the International Academy of Sex Research. For more than a decade, Tiefer had been working in the urology departments of New York hospitals, interviewing men who were being treated for sexual problems, conducting research and writing. She had soon become concerned that men's problems were being treated by the specialist urologists in a very mechanical way, and that sexual difficulties were being reduced to the quality of erections, divorced from the context of men's lives and relationships. In 1986, long before Viagra came along, she had published an article titled 'In Pursuit of the Perfect Penis', which sounded early warnings about what she saw as the medical takeover of male sexuality.[28]

With the arrival of Viagra, and Pfizer's entry into the field in the 1990s, Tiefer was soon foreseeing a powerful alliance emerging—a medicalisation of sexual difficulties driven by the medical profession and fuelled by pharmaceutical money. Her response to the rivers of funding starting to flow from drug companies was very different from Ray Rosen's. Her worry was that the small pools of sex researchers were in danger of being inundated by the muddy waters of drug company influence.[29] She was concerned that this might contract the focus of research on to the narrow, more physiological aspects of sexuality—like blood flow and hormones—for women as well as men. She'd heard that her old mate Ray Rosen was organising an important gathering on women's sexuality in Cape Cod, so she'd emailed him asking about the possibility of attending.

Rosen's reply to the request was blunt. The two were old friends so he felt he could be candid with her. He revealed that the main point of the meeting was to work out how to assess female sexual function in clinical trials involving drugs. In other words, the meeting would focus on how to measure the impacts of experimental drugs like Viagra on women. Perhaps even more importantly, his email revealed that the drug companies would be picking up the tab for the entire Cape Cod affair:

> The meeting is completely supported by pharmaceutical companies, and approximately half of the audience will be pharmaceutical representatives. The goal is to foster active and positive collaboration between the two groups. Only investigators who have experience with, or special interest in working collaboratively with the drug industry have been invited, and that's the obvious reason I had not included you. Your views of the issue are very well known to all.[30]

Rosen's email went on to offer Tiefer the chance to attend only if she was 'willing to genuinely participate' in the meeting, an offer she ultimately declined after much deliberation, deciding she did not want to be part of this emerging collaboration with industry. Others had no such reservations, and a core of sex experts and drug company officials soon flew into Cape Cod from across the United States and around the world.

That Cape Cod conference marks the dawning of the new era of 'active and positive' collaboration between the global pharmaceutical industry and a small group of highly influential sex researchers focused on women's sexual problems. Discussions at that meeting would help inform a whole new scientific agenda, ultimately sparking new research projects, surveys, questionnaires and educational programs—the very building blocks of the science of this new dysfunction. Most immediately it would lead to more meetings of sex researchers, many of which would be heavily sponsored by industry. The following year, a group of 'thought leaders', including Ray Rosen, would meet in Boston in a closed session to revise the definitions of female sexual dysfunction, or FSD. The vast majority of the nineteen 'thought leaders' would disclose that they had some sort of relationship with industry.[31] As in many areas of medicine, the drug companies weren't writing the definitions, but the panels of experts who did included many with financial ties to those companies. Typically, those ties could involve being an adviser or consultant, being contracted to do research or being paid for speaking engagements.

That important meeting, at which the definitions were revised, took place just up the road from Cape Cod in Boston, where another of Ray Rosen's colleagues, Dr Irwin Goldstein, was based. A professor of urology and gynaecology, Irwin Goldstein started his professional life as an engineer before switching to sex research, an area in which he is highly regarded and has become well recognised. A practising doctor and widely published university academic, Goldstein has also retained his boyish good looks along the way. In addition to all his publicly funded research via grants from the National Institutes of Health, Goldstein has worked with many of the world's biggest drug companies, which he sees as playing a paramount role in helping build the new science of sexual medicine.[32]

By the start of the twenty-first century, the gatherings of this group of researchers interested in women's sexual difficulties were becoming annual scientific conferences, now attracting support from more than twenty companies, with Pfizer as a key sponsor.[33] And the drug companies weren't just funding the get-togethers: on some occasions, their staff were actually attending as well, taking part inside the scientific sessions. These were the sorts of activities to which drug company research manager Darby Stephens was referring when she talked of working closely with 'thought leaders' to jointly develop this new disease entity. Yet while this close working relationship is the norm in medicine, not all drug company managers are as candid when it comes to describing it.[34] An official from Pfizer was far less forthcoming than Darby Stephens when he was interviewed about his company's activities. The way he told it, the giant corporation was simply playing a 'passive' role by providing unrestricted grants for conferences in response to requests from physicians. Importantly, he also referred to FSD as a 'disease'.[35]

More recently, Pfizer has described the grants it provides for conferences as part of a much broader process of partnering with medical, scientific and patient organisations, helping to 'strengthen communities' and produce a 'healthier world'. Confirming Irwin Goldstein's views about industry's paramount role, the world's biggest drug giant proudly states that it has conducted and sponsored many scientific studies in the field of FSD, not just testing drugs, but also generating knowledge about the 'nature of female sexual dysfunction and its impact on women and their partners'.[36]

The sponsored gatherings at Cape Cod and Boston weren't only a chance for informal socialising and an opportunity to build friendships between marketing managers and university-based researchers. They were also the places where the new science of sexual medicine was being constructed, the new corporate-sponsored knowledge was being created, and the latest definitions of FSD were being written. These gatherings can be highly influential in the wider world of medicine and among the general public. Deliberations at these meetings are often covered in the media, and later published as important journal articles or guidelines for treatment, which in turn can be carried dutifully to your doctor's door by friendly drug company sales reps eager to educate the medical profession about the latest disorders. Embedded in a lot of this material is a strong view that common sexual difficulties are best described as medical dysfunctions. The downstream impact of all this on your doctor and the way he or she thinks about the problems in your sex life cannot be overstated.

Within a few short years of the historic meeting in Cape Cod, the drug companies were funding far more than just conferences for sex specialists. They would hand out direct grants to universities to educate medical students about women's sexual health, fund educational seminars for practising doctors and workshops for healthcare journalists. In the case of Pfizer at least, some of their sales staff would also ply doctors with kickbacks and inducements, according to court documents from an official whistleblower.[37] All of this was long before any sex drug had even been approved for women. A key aim was to win widespread acceptance of the idea that a woman's common sexual difficulties might be the sign of a treatable dysfunction. For many researchers, all this activity was bringing what they regarded as long-overdue recognition to women's sexual suffering, and legitimacy to its study. For the drug companies, it was a strategic part of the planning for what was being billed as the next billion-dollar market.

A forward-looking business intelligence report in 2003 named FSD drugs as an area of great future growth for the pharmaceutical industry, part of the burgeoning 'lifestyle' market including medicines for baldness, smoking cessation and obesity.[38] The report was prepared for industry insiders and, with a hefty price tag, was never intended for public consumption. However, a leaked copy described how drug companies were 'expanding the patient pool' by using marketing campaigns to change public perceptions about things that used to be considered part of normal life. 'The medicalisation of many natural processes,' the report observed, 'is creating markets for lifestyle drugs for those who want to optimise quality of life.' It predicted that the market for FSD drugs could soon approach a billion dollars a year. The days when the treatment of sex problems was dominated by the idea that therapy could render sexual inadequacy obsolete were quickly forgotten, swept away in a collective enthusiasm for new panaceas to treat this new dysfunction, and the billions that might flow from it. But the enthusiasm was not universal.

Leonore Tiefer was by now pointing out in her writings that the post-sixties opportunities for the sexual emancipation of women were sadly being squandered in the medical takeover of sex.[39] Rather than attaining further freedom, the fear was that women were being subtly encouraged to feel inadequate, or even dysfunctional, if they failed to live up to a new unrealistic norm of a constant desire for sex. Right on cue, the new blue pill bounced straight from the doctor's surgery to the centre of popular culture. Viagra famously made a cameo appearance in the television series *Sex and the City*, when Samantha took the drug and apparently enhanced her already considerable sexual enthusiasm.[40] Apart from her broader social critique, Tiefer was also busy documenting drug company sponsorship of all the important meetings where the new disorders were being developed. The resulting evidence offered a rare insight into the extraordinary extent of pharmaceutical involvement with an emerging field of medicine.

Informed in part by this evidence, an article in the *British Medical Journal* (*BMJ*) described the making of FSD as the 'freshest, clearest example we have' of the corporate-sponsored creation of a disease.[41] The article caused media reaction around the world, and was heavily criticised by several 'thought leaders' in sex research. They felt it played down the genuine suffering of women with legitimate sexual difficulties and set back the aim of finding safe and effective treatments for them.

The *BMJ* piece also brought a negative response from Shere Hite, author of *The Hite Report*. She criticised it, but from a very different perspective. For her, it didn't go anywhere near far enough. Hite claimed that in the race to get a pill to market, the pharmaceutical industry was fundamentally misunderstanding women's sexuality due to serious flaws in the definitions being used. She argued that the four supposedly distinct disorders of FSD—desire, arousal, orgasm and pain—were in reality not independent of each other. 'Anticipating pain will kill off desire,' she wrote in a feisty opinion piece published internationally.[42]

'An arousal pill may be a costly waste of time if the root cause of that lack of arousal is not addressed.'

Hite's perspective, based on the material collected for her research, is that many difficulties aren't due to a dysfunction, but rather to the century-old misunderstanding of female sexual pleasure, dating back at least to Freud. A lack of orgasm during intercourse is a 'crucial and common underlying reason why many women become disenchanted and uninterested in sex', she argued, pointing out what other research also demonstrates: that many—maybe most—women don't reach orgasm regularly through intercourse alone. Yet the popularly accepted version of sex is still focused squarely on intercourse as the time when both partners reach the climax of their sexual pleasure. 'It is not women who need to change, or be made different through drugs, but the drug industry's outdated notion of how couples should have sex,' wrote Hite, echoing debates about the site of female sexual pleasure that had been bouncing back and forwards down through the decades of the previous century.

The notion that both partners in a heterosexual relationship can consistently come to climax simply through intercourse will sound awfully old-fashioned to some readers. Certainly many women can and do reach orgasm through intercourse. But since Kinsey, and indeed even before, the early science of sexuality was confirming that, for many women, the clitoris was the site of their orgasm, and that vaginal intercourse alone was not routinely going to bring all women to climax. Yet so much popular culture seemingly hasn't caught up with the facts. How many sex scenes in highly regarded films still replay an outdated version of love-making based primarily and solely on intercourse? Try to name a few Hollywood blockbusters, or even art-house features, that accurately portray the physical reality of female orgasm. Even in much supposedly sophisticated pornography, according to Hite, clitoral stimulation is used only as a warm-up, and is not portrayed to the point of climax. For her, the dominant form of sex—even in the twenty-first century—is one that still puts male orgasm before female orgasm, reflecting the still subservient position of women in society as a whole: 'It's not arousal pills we need, but a whole new kind of physical relations with each other.'

Exposing the uncertainty and debate around whether women's common sexual problems are best classified as *dysfunctions* or *difficulties* is not an attempt to trivialise them. On the contrary, the hope is that doctors will diagnose women, and offer them therapies, only when they really require them, rather than because a powerful drug company that is funding their education wants to see tens of millions of women labelled in order to open the doors to a new mass market. Labelling a woman with a medical condition when she mightn't actually have one can mean failing to get to the root of her problem—especially if it is not her problem alone but has arisen from her relationship. A wrong diagnosis and potentially unnecessary medications can carry harms and costs for the individual woman involved, as well as for those footing the bill for national health budgets, already straining under the weight of too much medicine.[43]

Much of the building of the science of this new dysfunction has happened in the light shining out from that 1997 meeting in Cape Cod, where Ray Rosen so successfully helped to bring together the doctors and the drug companies. Another big milestone was laid down less than two years later in 1999, when a landmark article appeared in one of the world's leading medical journals. The article in the *Journal of the American Medical Association* reported on the results of a large sex survey.[44] It stated baldly that 43 per cent of women suffered from some form of sexual dysfunction, and that this was an important public health concern. As we'll soon discover, the big figure sparked an even bigger reaction. But here was the next building block in the foundation for the new disease that Darby Stephens and her colleagues and competitors in the industry were rushing to help develop.

Two

43 per cent

[T]he total prevalence of sexual dysfunction . . . for women . . . 43% . . . an important public health concern.

—*Journal of the American Medical Association, 1999*

Let us be absolutely clear here. The article in the *Journal of the American Medical Association* that famously featured the 43 per cent figure[1] gave birth to one of the most pervasive medical myths of our time. The claim flowing from the article—that there is a condition called 'female sexual dysfunction' requiring treatment and affecting one in every two women—is an exaggeration as extreme as it is absurd. The evidence assembled in the article never supported such an assertion, as even its lead author attests, yet different versions of this claim have been shouted far and wide ever since. Since its publication in 1999, the influential journal article has been cited by other scientific papers more than 1000 times, and in the wider culture on tens of thousands of occasions.[2]

'Bad news in the bedroom, a sex study finds widespread sexual dysfunction', screeched one popular magazine when the journal article first appeared.[3] A management consultancy firm excitedly pointed out that, with 43 per cent of women suffering from this 'treatable disease', there must be an awful lot of 'unmet need', and the 'sexual dysfunction market' would offer great opportunities for companies that sell therapies.[4] The 43 per cent figure worked its way from scientific journals into medical textbooks and magazine articles all over the world, becoming part of the scientific bedrock for this new disease. Yet no matter how many times the statistic is repeated, it doesn't make the claim of a medical condition affecting one in every two women any more accurate or any less misleading. The way such figures can come to be so influential is a fascinating part of the story of how modern diseases are made, and FSD is the latest example we have. So where better to start this part of the tale than on a Wednesday in February 1999, the day this 43 per cent figure first emerged into the glare of global publicity.

Ed Laumann's striking blue eyes shine out at you from his strong sincere face, fringed these days by his shining white hair. The professor of sociology from Chicago University has had a long research interest in human sexuality. He even holds the distinction of having had the US government try to shut down public funding for some of his work. A number of politicians were morally objecting to a large sex survey Laumann had wanted to run, back in the days when conservatives were still in the political ascendency in Washington. His sex survey eventually went ahead with funding from philanthropic foundations, and the results were published in a book in the early 1990s.[5] Several years later, a selected portion of those survey results would be re-published in detail in the *Journal of the American Medical Association*, with Edward O. Laumann listed as first author.

The sociologist is particularly proud of the original survey, which was based on a large national sample of interviews with over 3000 Americans. It has, in fact, been highly praised as one of the first to use modern statistical methods of 'probability sampling'. That's the method used to try to gather a truly representative group of people in order to give a reliable picture of a whole nation's sexuality. Alfred Kinsey's famous interviews with more than 10 000 men and women, while historic, did not employ those same sampling methods, and his findings have been criticised for not being representative.

When the HIV epidemic hit in the 1980s, Kinsey's work (despite its limitations) was still one of the most comprehensive surveys of American sexual behaviour. Clearly there was a desperate need to update the knowledge and learn more about the sexual behaviour of Americans, hence the motivation for Laumann's survey. As it turned out, the study found lower rates of homosexuality than Kinsey did; unsurprisingly, it also discovered that a person's chances of catching a sexually transmitted infection went up dramatically as the number of sexual partners increased.

While the main focus of the national sex study was about trying to better understand and fight HIV/AIDS, it included almost as a sideline some questions about sexual difficulties. Among many other items in the hour-and-a-half-long survey interview, the staff working with Ed Laumann asked women a quick series of simple questions about whether they'd experienced any of seven common difficulties for several months or more during the past year. The questions asked things like whether they'd lacked interest in sex, felt anxious about their sexual performance, had trouble with lubrication, failed to orgasm, came to orgasm too quickly or experienced pain on intercourse. By simply answering yes to just one of these questions, women were then categorised as having a sexual dysfunction. When they were all added up, the number of women in this category reached 43 per cent. And this is the source of the 43 per cent statistic that appeared in the aforementioned article, which has become part of the foundation for a global campaign claiming almost half of all women suffer with a sexual dysfunction that might be treatable with powerful drugs.

The obvious problem is that common difficulties are being confused with medical dysfunctions—a confusion that occurs time and time again with surveys of this condition.[6] The 43 per cent result came from simply adding up the numbers of women answering yes to a simple question about their experiences, no matter how serious they were. Women were classified as having sexual dysfunction if they answered 'yes' to just one of these questions, even if the answer to the other six questions was no. The questions did not ask if they had a mild or severe problem, or whether women had a little or a lot of trouble with lubrication. In the totals from this survey (and in others) researchers are including women with passing problems that might be best seen as healthy adaptive responses to life circumstances. Their findings are estimates of the numbers of people with common experiences; they are not estimates of the numbers of women whose situations are so severe and distressing they may warrant the diagnosis of a medical condition.

Importantly, since at least 1998 the conventional view among those who have been promoting a more medical approach to FSD has been that a woman must be *distressed* by her situation before she can qualify for a diagnosis.[7] Yet the original survey questions made no mention of distress. As it turns out, the 1999 journal article actually carried a small but very significant caveat to its findings. It noted, almost in passing, that its results were 'not equivalent to clinical diagnosis' of dysfunction. Unfortunately, caveats like this have too often been lost in the gold rush to build this lucrative new condition.

Impressive statistics like 43 per cent can serve very important roles. Being able to throw around enormous estimates of the prevalence of a medical condition directly helps drug companies to claim there is a gaping 'unmet need' for their new products. It also helps researchers to attract the attention of funding bodies, and patient advocacy groups to generate interest from journalists keen for a dramatic headline. In short, these figures help bring the recognition each field of medicine so desperately seems to want—and specialists working in this new field of sexual medicine are no exception.[8]

One of the key textbooks about women's sexual dysfunction actually makes a direct reference to the critical importance of the 43 per cent figure. On page 745 of *Women's Sexual Function and Dysfunction*, the editors acknowledge concerns that such large figures may give the appearance that ordinary life experiences are being portrayed as the signs of a medical condition.[9] Yet, according to the editors of this textbook, the survey that produced the 43 per cent statistic has proved very beneficial in 'spreading the word' about sexual dysfunction to those women who qualify for a clinical diagnosis. At the same time though, the inflated nature of the statistic has helped create a strong backlash. Leonore Tiefer, like many others in the field, rejects the claim that 43 per cent of women suffer with a dysfunction, and sees the figure as being extremely unhelpful. But she says with her trademark sense of humour that she finds the 760-page textbook very useful around the office, not least because its size is just right for doing upper body exercises!

Another of those concerned about the size of the 43 per cent figure has been psychologist Dr Sandra Leiblum. She has argued that genuine dysfunction among women is less common than 43 per cent, and that the statistic has contributed to an over-medicalisation of women's sexual experiences. 'I think there is dissatisfaction and perhaps disinterest among a lot of women, but that doesn't mean they have a disease,' she said in an interview in 2002.[10] Dr Irwin Goldstein, one of the editors of *Women's Sexual Function and Dysfunction*, has dismissed suggestions from his colleague that the 43 per cent may indicate the prevalence of difficulties rather than real dysfunction. 'I love psychologists,' he told a reporter, 'but they don't deal with evidence.'

Back in February 1999, it wasn't long before Ed Laumann's pleasure about his latest publication was turning into an experience more akin to pain. Just four days after publication, a major piece appeared in the *New York Times*. The *Times* was reporting that the *Journal of the American Medical Association* had failed to reveal that two authors of the 43 per cent article had some sort of financial relationship with the pharmaceutical giant Pfizer.[11] One of those authors was Ed Laumann. As the *Times* pointed out, the journal article did find that many common sexual problems had social and emotional roots, which drugs couldn't do much about. But the journal article had also called for the development of 'appropriate therapies' for the vast numbers of supposedly dysfunctional women. Those therapies could potentially include counselling and drugs—in particular Pfizer's Viagra, which had just been approved for men and was at that time actively being studied in women. In other words, Pfizer stood to benefit greatly from the article's findings of an enormous potential market among women—a great 'unmet need'. Therefore, any connection between the article's authors and the company represented the sort of conflict of interest that should have been disclosed, but hadn't been.

Pfizer had not funded the original national survey, nor had it had anything to do with the later rewriting of results. However, Ed Laumann had joined one of Pfizer's advisory committees in the lead-up to the launch of Viagra, and that fact was not disclosed in the article. The second author, whose conflicts of interest were similarly not disclosed, was Ray Rosen, the psychologist who'd organised that crucial meeting between drug companies and sex researchers at Cape Cod just a year or so earlier. Two months after the 43 per cent article first appeared, an embarrassing correction was published by the *Journal of the American Medical Association*. In tiny print, it was disclosed that Laumann had served on Pfizer's committee, and that Rosen had worked as a consultant or received research support from a total of five drug companies, including Pfizer.[12]

According to Ed Laumann, the idea for the 1999 journal article focusing on the prevalence of sexual dysfunction in men and woman had come from Rosen in the first place. 'Ray suggested it to me,' Laumann said. He explained that Rosen used to quote the statistics from the earlier book of survey results, but that a short article in a big journal might be a better way of making people more widely aware of them. Dr Rosen declined to answer questions for this book, so it is unclear how he sees the background to the famous paper or the controversy and criticism surrounding the infamous 43 per cent figure. Ed Laumann, however, was happy to chat about both subjects, over morning tea at a big drug company-funded sex conference in Paris a decade later, in the exhibit hall just across the way from the Pfizer stand.

So what did the sociologist think about the way that 43 per cent statistic had been used to represent an estimate of the numbers of women with a medical dysfunction? 'That's clearly a misrepresentation,' Laumann said with evident frustration. 'First of all I don't think that these things are medical dysfunctions, in the sense that they should require active intervention.' And how did he feel about his figures being used as an indication of the size of the market of women who might need drugs? 'The problem is you can't really control how people are going to spin numbers,' he responded, adding that it would be a mistake to see 43 per cent of women as a potential market for medicines: 'It's like dangling a huge carrot out there to say, just look at all those people, half the population, ready to gobble some kind of solution, medication or something like that. It's a lack of understanding of what it is that really drives those numbers. And what drives the numbers is stress, physical and social stress, exhaustion, not being in a relationship with somebody you care about, so you're not sexually interested.'[13]

The Chicago sociologist has clearly been stung by the heated controversy surrounding this work and the repeated criticism of the 43 per cent figure. In subsequent articles, he's been careful to make his caveats more prominent. In a chapter in *Women's Sexual Function and Dysfunction*, Ed Laumann and a colleague analysed the results of fifteen surveys designed to ascertain how many women have the condition. They came up with some scathing criticisms of their own about the way in which common difficulties uncovered during these surveys are often portrayed. 'Despite widespread usage of the term "sexual dysfunction",' they wrote, 'most of these studies rely not on clinical diagnosis of dysfunction, but on self-reports of symptoms or sexual problems.'[14]

Laumann went on to emphasise that in almost all the surveys carried out, the high rates of sexual problems apparently being uncovered did not equate to rates of medical dysfunction that might be diagnosed according to the technical definitions. One of the only studies to actually try to find out how many men and women in the population suffered from a diagnosable dysfunction came up with a rate of just 3 per cent. In a sense, Laumann was drawing attention to the inflated estimates of this condition, alerting us all to the myth that has arisen—ironically, partly from one of his own journal articles.

Echoing a wider concern expressed by others, he also criticised the surveys for trying to look at an *individual* woman's sexual difficulties in isolation from the context of her *relationships*. 'Many studies assessed the prevalence of problems with desire, arousal, orgasm and pain without investigating the nature of the corresponding sexual relationships,' he wrote in his review. Perhaps most importantly, the sociology professor raised the awkward issue of how to define a sexual problem. He pointed out that what was missing in many studies and surveys was 'whether the respondent views a particular symptom as a problem'. In other words, leaving aside the inflated estimates of dysfunction, how many of the millions of woman who supposedly have sexual problems—according to these survey findings—are in fact experiencing something they consider to be a genuine problem at all?

This is a question well worth pondering for a moment. When we look behind the claims of high rates of sexual dysfunction—like 43 per cent—it becomes clearer that the studies have actually come up with estimates of the rates of common 'difficulties'—if they can even be called that. But looking more closely, how many of these common experiences—like a lack of interest in sex, troubles with lubrication, or coming to orgasm *too quickly*—are even seen as problems by the women experiencing them? And if she does look on them as a problem, does she see them primarily as her own personal problem, or rather something to do with her relationship or her partner? As others have observed, the criteria used by researchers to identify a sexual problem are arbitrary and don't necessarily relate to the reality of women's lives.[15]

The same year Ed Laumann's paper was published another sex survey was being set up, organised by a team working in Bloomington, Indiana. This time the survey was being run by the Kinsey Institute, the outfit named after the celebrated sex researcher. Continuing the work Kinsey and his colleagues had conducted decades earlier, the Institute's general approach is to view the inhibition of women's sexual response as an adaptive mechanism. Under this approach, a woman's lack of interest in sex may well be an appropriate and understandable reaction to life circumstances—stress, tiredness or threatening patterns of behaviour from a partner—rather than a sign of some medical malfunction.

Smaller than Laumann's, this next survey involved almost 1000 American women. It was overseen by Kinsey Institute director Dr John Bancroft,[16] a respected sex researcher and one of the people who had great concerns about this new claim that 43 per cent of women had a sexual dysfunction. Bancroft believed the term 'dysfunction' could be highly misleading, making many women feel they had a malfunction when they did not. As to the figure of 43 per cent, Bancroft felt it was outrageous, and did not stand up scientifically.[17] Further, he argued, the statistic was being used wrongly as evidence of a widespread need for medical treatments, including drugs, even though Laumann's journal article itself had shown that sexual problems were commonly linked to relationship issues and other quality of life concerns. Bancroft was worried that, in the era of Viagra, the complexity of female sexuality might be reduced to narrow questions of how much blood was flowing to a woman's genitals.

The Kinsey Institute survey asked women a range of questions about their sexuality, their relationships and their physical responses during sex, including questions about lubrication, pain and orgasm. The study found that 24 per cent of women expressed distress about their sexual relationships and/or their own sexuality. Drilling down to what might be causing this widespread dissatisfaction, the survey results suggested the state of a woman's emotional well-being, and her feelings about her relationship with her partner during sexual activity, were more important determinants of her distress than problems around physical arousal, lubrication or orgasm.

The survey results also indicated that distress about sex did not increase with age, even though interest in sex might decline. This reinforced other evidence suggesting that getting older might bring a slowing of sexual interest or activity, but it also generally means less likelihood of worrying about it.[18] Like others, Bancroft was alarmed that portraying common problems as dysfunctions—as he believed the *Journal of the American Medical Association* article had done—could make many older women think there was something wrong with them when there wasn't. 'While it is good to encourage older couples to maintain and foster their sexual intimacy,' he wrote, 'should we be encouraging older women to regard themselves as "dysfunctional" because they have less sexual interest than when they were younger?'[19]

Here is a reaffirmation of Kinsey's celebration of the enormous variation in human sexuality. It is a call to acknowledge the ebbs and flows of sexual life rather than manufacture new medical conditions where the sexual activity of the young becomes the norm for all, and we label those who don't measure up as abnormal or dysfunctional. Bancroft's comments are part of a broader concern that the changes in sexuality that tend to happen naturally as we age are being reframed, or re-imagined, as a health or medical problem requiring treatment.[20] Yet, at the same time, his perspective readily accepts that some sexual difficulties can be severe and long lasting, and that a medical approach may sometimes be entirely necessary. Criticising the drug companies for trying to portray common sexual problems as treatable disorders doesn't mean rejecting the obvious benefits of a medical approach and medicines, when needed. For John Bancroft, himself a medical doctor, some malfunctioning in a woman's sexual response could occur because of the side-effects of a drug, because she was suffering a disease like cancer or because of some failure of her healthy adaptive mechanisms. In such cases, in his view, the word 'dysfunction' may well be appropriate, and treatments valuable, including medicines proven to be safe and effective.[21] Like many surveys, the one conducted by the Kinsey Institute was funded by the pharmaceutical industry, and in this case the company—Eli Lilly—had also hired Bancroft as a consultant.

The journal article based on the results of that survey was published in mid-2003, and by the end of that year Lilly's sex drug Cialis would be approved for men. Like Viagra, this drug acts by enhancing blood flow to the genitals—a physiological process the industry hoped would help some of the many millions of women said to have this new dysfunction. Yet as the industry was becoming excited by the profitable possibilities, respected voices like Bancroft and Tiefer were raising questions about whether there really was a mass market of women with a medical condition requiring drug treatment. If distressing sexual difficulties were largely caused by relationship and emotional factors, rather than a medical dysfunction of poor blood flow, where on earth was this market for drugs?

John Bancroft was asking two very pointed questions: When might a dysfunction better be called a difficulty? And when was a difficulty better seen as normal life anyway? His journal article analysed the ways in which several other influential surveys had dealt with these awkward questions. He concluded that many of the women supposedly found to have sexual problems through sex surveys often didn't even regard themselves as having problems or weren't distressed by them. In other words, surveys were not only confusing difficulties with dysfunctions; they might have even been finding problems where none existed. Which begs another awkward question: to what extent are these surveys, which often generate a lot of coverage in the media, actually helping to paint a picture of a new epidemic of sexual difficulties that may not in fact be there in the first place?

Bancroft went so far as to suggest that until there was an agreed way to accurately define whether a woman had a problem with her sexuality or not, running big surveys to assess how widespread they were was a 'hazardous' activity. He also called for a whole new approach to assessing sexual problems, in which a woman's own description of her experience is seen as more important, 'rather than her answers to questions based on pre-conceived concepts of female dysfunction'.

Just a few short months later, that call for a new approach to assessing sexual concerns was heard and heeded on the other side of the Atlantic Ocean. A British team based in London decided to take the radical step of conducting a sex survey that included questions asking women straight up whether they thought they had a sexual problem.[22] The plan was to try to find out how many women might end up with a label of dysfunction if their doctors used a standard approach, and compare that with the number of women who actually saw themselves as having a sexual problem. The researchers recruited 400 women from several general practices across London. The research project was unusual, and its methods rather complicated, but they went something like this.

In order to see how many women might be diagnosed by their doctor under a medical approach, the researchers used a questionnaire and a definition of sexual dysfunction derived from an international manual of diseases used in Britain— similar to the American *DSM*. (A key difference between the British and US definitions is whether or not the woman must experience distress. In the British definition, this requirement is absent.) Unlike other studies of this kind, the British researchers also asked the women directly whether they thought they had any sexual problem, even of a mild nature, and how distressing that problem might be. In addition, the women were asked whether they considered their problem to be a medical one— like arthritis—an emotional one or relationship related—like a lack of time together with a partner. The findings were stunning.

When the researchers looked at the results from the questionnaire used to assess the women, they found that a whopping 38 per cent might qualify for a doctor's diagnosis of sexual dysfunction. But that figure then fell to 18 per cent if the woman herself was required to think she had a problem. When it was also required that the woman saw her problem as distressing, the figure fell again—this time to just 6 per cent, a world away from 38 per cent.

In other words, only a tiny proportion of women who were 'diagnosed' with a sexual dysfunction during this study saw themselves as having a sexual problem that distressed them. This is clearly only one small study with an unusual scientific approach, but it raises fascinating questions about the value of the definitions of these conditions. If only a very small number of women labelled as dysfunctional actually see themselves as having distressing sexual problems, what does that say about the definitions of the dysfunction? A major reality check is surely looming.

As to what the women saw as the origin of their sexual problems, the innovative London study found relationship and emotional issues were the most commonly perceived causes. For almost two-thirds of the women in the study who said they had a problem, difficulty with their relationship was seen as one of the factors. This doesn't mean those difficulties aren't genuine, but it does raise doubts about the relevance of drugs in treating them. Echoing the approaches of John Bancroft and Leonore Tiefer, the British researchers concluded that 'reduced sexual interest or response in women often appears to be an adaptation to stress or an unsatisfactory relationship. Many such adaptations may be short term and not classifiable as dysfunction.' This is a point of view shared by a lot of sex researchers who are uneasy about using the word 'dysfunction' to describe common problems.[23] 'Most women regard their sexual problems as something to do with relationships,' said Dr Michael King, the professor based at University College who oversaw the London survey and a psychiatrist with an interest in psychosexual medicine who regularly sees both male and female patients. 'I find very disturbing the drive to find a pill to medicalise everything to do with sex.'[24]

Unlike other studies of women's sexual problems, this British research was entirely free of pharmaceutical industry funding, and none of the researchers had any connections to any company. Michael King is one of the small but most likely growing numbers of doctors around the world who has decided not to accept any more free lunches from companies trying to woo his favour. He avoids financial relationships with them, and he's banned them from sponsoring meals in his medical school department. 'I'm not anti-pharmaceutical companies,' he says. 'They are incredibly important. I just don't like researchers getting so close to them.' While he fully recognises the need for doctors to work with drug companies testing drugs, he's worried when they join forces to conduct surveys or develop diagnostic tools, because of the potential that the marketing and the science will get mixed up. On a positive note, he argues that with all the attention drugs like Viagra are producing, people are more likely to be open with their doctors, even though they don't necessarily see their sexual problems as medical ones. Importantly, he points out that 'they are still afraid to talk to each other'. He is hinting that a frank conversation with one's sexual partner may often help a lot.

While Michael King might choose to avoid pharmaceutical companies' free lunches and financial ties, other researchers, however, very happily continue to work with industry on surveys of this condition. And sometimes the drug companies don't just fund the studies: they actively initiate them, run them and help write up their results. When sociologist Ed Laumann published the results of a later survey of sexual problems, this time around it was global—and this time it was directly funded by Pfizer.[25]

Funding wasn't where the company's role ended, either. One of the people who helped analyse and interpret the results was actually a Pfizer employee. And as Laumann explained it, the motivation for the huge international survey actually came from within Pfizer, which orchestrated it and paid for it. 'It was a marketing effort,' said Laumann bluntly, to help the drug company 'gauge the scale of interest' across the markets of many different nations.[26]

That study surveyed close to 30 000 men and women in almost 30 countries. It used similar questions to the ones Laumann had used in his original American survey, although this time round the results were not presented as dysfunctions, but rather as sexual problems. The rates were again extremely high, with findings that in some parts of the world over 40 per cent of women had experienced some problems. As an example, according to the results from countries in Northern Europe, almost 20 per cent of women apparently had the problem of failing to reach orgasm, with that figure rising to over 40 per cent in Southeast Asia. Those statistics sound horrifyingly high, and they give the sense the world is living through a plague of sexual problems. But it is worth taking a closer look at how those figures were calculated.

A more detailed examination of the results of the Pfizer-funded study reveals that the estimates like 40 per cent were in fact the grand total. Unlike his original US survey, which had only asked a 'yes/no' question, this time round the global survey asked a follow-up question. If women said yes to having had a particular experience, they were then asked to judge how often they had it—occasionally, periodically or frequently. The totals were obtained by including all women who experienced that problem, no matter how often. So if you focus only on those women who failed to reach orgasm 'frequently', for example, the dramatic estimates collapse in Northern Europe from almost 20 per cent down to just 4 per cent. In Southeast Asia, the numbers fall from over 40 per cent to just 7 per cent.[27]

Similarly, for the problem described as 'lacking interest in sex', the sponsored survey found a rate of 30 per cent in Southern Europe and over 40 per cent in the Middle East. But again, when you exclude women with occasional or periodic difficulties and just look at those women who lacked interest 'frequently', the figures fall to just 8 per cent in Europe and to 11 per cent in the Middle East. In their analysis of the factors associated with sexual problems, Laumann's team themselves excluded women who had reported only 'occasional' problems.

Turning to the causes, this global study found that a woman's age had little impact on her sexual problems. The only exception to this, where age was an important factor, was in the area of lubrication difficulties, which unsurprisingly were also more common for those women who weren't having frequent sex.[28] It also found mental health issues were relevant, and that stresses from financial situations were associated with difficulties reaching orgasm, confirming the importance of life context. Once again, relationship factors affected the likelihood of sexual problems. For its part Pfizer sees the global survey as an important part of the work the company has done trying to 'understand the causes and nature of female sexual dysfunction and its impact on women and their partners'.[29]

While Pfizer was funding its international study, another big company racing to market a sex drug for women, Procter & Gamble (P&G), was funding its own global survey. According to the results of that survey, up to one in ten post-menopausal women suffered from a condition of low libido called 'hypoactive sexual desire disorder', or HSDD, one of the four disorders of FSD.[30] Women said to suffer with this condition happened to be the target market for P&G's testosterone drug, approved in Europe soon after the company's survey was published. In this case, the company not only funded the scientific survey, but a majority of those involved with writing up the results were company employees. Another was Ray Rosen, continuing the 'active and positive' collaboration with industry that he'd foreshadowed in the lead-up to that historic Cape Cod meeting.

Let's stop and try and work out what's been happening here. Powerful global companies are funding—and in some cases even orchestrating—scientific surveys that purport to show the extent of the problems their drugs are designed to treat. These surveys can sometimes attract media interest, get picked up by company-sponsored advocacy groups and even capture the attention of those in government. In summary, they can be extremely influential in creating a sense of a massive unmet need for new treatments. Yet when you pull back from the fine details of each individual survey, and start to take a bird's eye view of what's going on, certain patterns start to become clearer. Before a corporation unleashes its latest blockbuster solution, it tends to fund a survey that helps describe the size of the problem. And if the Americans can do it, so too can the German Boehringer, the company hoping to sell an old anti-depressant as the fix for women said to have the disorder of low desire, HSDD.

When the German company sent out a press release explaining that up to one in ten women suffer from HSDD, it cited a new survey in a scientific journal to back up its claim.[31] Not only did the company fund that survey, but all five authors had financial ties to the company. One of the authors was a company employee, and the lead author was a company consultant.

There's no suggestion any of these researchers on any of these surveys were fudging statistics in order to deliberately exaggerate the size of potential markets for their sponsors. The truth is, as others have pointed out, difficulties—even distressing ones—traditionally have been confused with diagnosable medical disorders, and it appeared that this tradition was continuing. These surveys tend to use just a few questions similar to the ones Laumann originally used and then tally up the results to produce alarmingly high totals, like one in ten women suffering from HSDD, which translates into tens of millions of women worldwide.

Some of the estimates you'll see and hear are literally so high they're laughable. A chapter in another textbook written by big names in the field, including Dr Irwin Goldstein, opened with this startling statement: 'Current data reveal that up to 76% of women have some sort of sexual dysfunction.'[32] An article in a leading Australian medical journal suggested the disorder of low desire may affect up to 50 per cent of women. Inflated as they may be, the figures help reinforce the impression that we are living with some kind of hidden scourge at which we must throw everything we can, including powerful pharmaceuticals.

Sexual medicine is, of course, not the only field where large estimates of disease numbers are regularly thrown around. One in eight of us supposedly has *social anxiety disorder*, one in five is said to have *irritable bowel syndrome*, and in any given year we're told a third of us have a mental illness.[33] Some have even claimed that one in five people suffers *motivational deficiency disorder*—a new condition announced to the world on 1 April 2006.[34] Such exaggerated claims have become a key feature of a medical landscape dominated by a pharmaceutical industry seeking ever-expanding markets. The figures would be funny if the harmful and wasteful consequences of unnecessary drug use weren't so deadly serious. But such huge estimates of the numbers of people suffering all these syndromes and sicknesses have helped spark a backlash of common sense. When it comes to claims that 43 per cent of women suffer with a sexual dysfunction, a large dose of healthy scepticism is just what the doctor ordered. Some researchers are happy to continue claiming this dysfunction is widespread, but others are using very different language.

When an Australian team wrote up the results of its sex survey of almost 20 000 people, it found an overwhelming majority were happy with their physical relationships, and that most people—both men and women—wanted more sex than they were having.[35] In addition, almost one in five women said they'd been forced or frightened into unwanted sex at some point in their lives, with half of that group having such an experience before the age of seventeen. When it came to sexual problems, the team found a large proportion of men, and even more women, experienced some sort of difficulty—whether it was a lack of interest in sex, vaginal dryness or pain on intercourse. However, the Australian researchers were very clear about interpreting these results, making sure they didn't unnecessarily exaggerate the nature of the problems, or describe them as the signs of a medical condition: 'We did not measure sexual dysfunction and we would strongly caution against any attempt to read our data in that way.'[36] The Australian study was publicly funded, without any sponsorship or involvement from the pharmaceutical industry.

The researchers also noted that they were unsure how many of the experiences that they'd classified as sexual difficulties were actually seen as problems by the people experiencing them. To shed more light on this issue, in a more recent study a new follow-up question was added to the original list of questions about sexual difficulties. For example, if a woman answered yes to having had a period of lacking interest in sex, she was then asked whether she considered this to be a major problem. The results were dramatic, but perhaps not so surprising. Fewer than one in ten of the women who had said they experienced a lack of interest in sex described this as a major problem for them.

A senior member of that Australian survey team was Dr Juliet Richters, who works at the University of New South Wales in Sydney. A specialist in the social aspects of sexual health, rather than a medical doctor, she says she doesn't come from a tradition that sees everything as a disease. From her perspective, most sexual difficulties are not physical dysfunctions to be fixed with pharmaceuticals, but instead 'failures to meet social rules of sexual behaviour'.[37] In other words, for whatever reason, a lot of people feel they're not living up to the social norms expected of them.

To illustrate what she means, Richters proposed we do a short exercise, using the famous seven questions that produced the infamous 43 per cent estimate of female sexual dysfunction. The questions used in the original survey asked women whether they had lacked interest in having sex, been unable to reach orgasm, or felt anxious about their ability to perform. To make her point, Juliet Richters suggested turning the questions into instructions: 'you should be constantly interested in having sex; you should be able to reach orgasm every time; you should not feel anxious about your ability to perform sexually'.[38] These, she believes, are the social rules of sexual behaviour that sit below the survey questions being put to women. In her view, it is illogical to treat a failure to obey a rule as a dysfunction. The exercise has its limitations, but it shows that there are very different ways of trying to understand sexual difficulties and dissatisfactions. It also shows there are lots of sex researchers across the world who don't see common ups and downs as the symptoms of disorders to be potentially treated with drugs. Further still, it helps demonstrate that the questions we ask determine the answers we get, which is why some researchers interested in women's sexual problems are looking for new sorts of questions.

As part of the work for her PhD thesis, a young British researcher named Kirstin Mitchell assembled and analysed many of the important and influential surveys of sexual dysfunction published around the world. One of her conclusions was that sex surveys 'often confuse self-reported problems with medically diagnosable disorders', echoing previous comments by Ed Laumann.[39] Mitchell also raised doubts about a lot of the highly inflated results, arguing that for a survey's findings to be valuable in public health terms it should avoid including women with passing problems and those whose difficulties are an adaptive response to their situation. Like others, she's emphasised that many sexual problems are related strongly to life events such as relationship difficulties, work stresses or simply having young kids in the house, and they shouldn't be misrepresented as medical dysfunctions.

In relation to the seven questions used to produce the 43 per cent claim, Kirstin Mitchell has pointed out that while they appear acceptable, they have not been subject to scientific testing. In other words, the seven questions were not actually proven scientifically to be a reliable way of getting to the bottom of what is going wrong for women sexually. And that's exactly what Dr Mitchell has been trying to do. She's been designing a new tool for use in the general population that she hopes will better get at the problems women themselves believe they're facing, rather than working with a construct of 'sexual dysfunction' that may not match well with the reality for many women. She is doing it as part of a team based at the London School of Hygiene and Tropical Medicine, without any funding from drug companies.

What is perhaps most frightening about the surveys estimating how widespread these disorders are is not the inflated findings that millions of women are affected; rather, it is the sheer enormity of the global misunderstanding of the nature and size of this purported medical problem. You may not have heard the results of any of these surveys yet, but as the pharmaceutical marketing machinery starts working in your town or city you certainly will. Despite the criticism that they confuse difficulties with dysfunctions, their big headline findings pack a punch and they will have an impact. The claim that 43 per cent of women suffer from a treatable sexual dysfunction may have been heavily attacked—some would say discredited—but it has apparently also proved highly valuable in 'spreading the word' about this new condition and it is still being used. Without denying some women do face genuine problems, it seems time to ask whether these surveys and their big statistics may be helping to create the impression of an epidemic of disease where none exists, and whether sponsors are helping to manufacture the unmet need their drugs might later treat.

But before you can start to treat a new disease, you need new tools to diagnose it in the doctor's surgery and, in order to see how well your treatments are working, new ways to measure women's pleasure.

Three

Measuring pleasure

... a new, easy to use five-question diagnostic tool ... the Decreased Sexual Desire Screener (DSDS) enables clinicians who are not necessarily experts in female sexual dysfunction to diagnose the condition with high accuracy in a few minutes.

—Drug company press release, Germany

A woman is taken into a small room, where she's given a pair of futuristic video glasses to wear. The lights are dimmed, the surround-sound pumps into her ears and the images of an erotic video begin to flash before her eyes. There's a vibrator there if the woman wants to use it and some instructions if she doesn't know how. A short time later, another person will quietly enter the darkened room and proceed, as discreetly as possible, to place a small, hard object gently against the woman's clitoris. This is not a high-tech peep show for girls, but a form of diagnostic testing in a commercial medical clinic, the twenty-first century temple of scientific technology. Here the high priests and priestesses of sexual medicine are trying to measure women's pleasure with ultrasound probes testing the flow of blood to their genitals.

With soaring sales of the new drug Viagra pumping penises and profits, by the early 2000s anticipation was soon spilling over at the possibilities of a sex pill for women. If this apparently widespread condition called female sexual dysfunction was due in part to poor blood flow, and there was a drug that might be able to fix it, then there was clearly an urgent need to start testing women. And that's exactly what new sex clinics soon began to do.

'Blood flow problems are probably under-recognised as a contributor to sexual dysfunction in woman,' said one health professional, giving the media a tour of a new state of the art clinic. The clinic took a holistic multidisciplinary approach— including yoga, counselling and pills—to the treatment of sexual dysfunction, which it claimed on its website affected 43 per cent of women.[1] On the day of the clinic's opening, the doctor explained how the erotic videos and ultrasound machines would be used to try to measure whether a woman had 'normal' blood flow, an aspect of sexuality said to have become more important than we used to realise. 'We're on the frontier of a huge new field of medicine here,' she offered enthusiastically.

Out on that medical frontier there's a race to diagnose the one in two women, the 43 per cent, said by some to be suffering silently with this condition. Yet, there is little agreement about the best way to go about that diagnosing. In their attempts to measure pleasure some doctors have started probing into women's most intimate sexual spaces. In the clinics and the research labs, they've been testing everything from the flow of blood to the clitoris to the levels of testosterone in that blood, from the chemical reactions in the brain to the sexual chemistry in the bedroom. There are the ultrasound machines and the probes pressed to the clitoris, high-tech tampons for the aroused vagina, and little clips that take the temperature of the labia.[2] In addition, some researchers are looking for testosterone 'deficiencies', and using scans to find abnormalities in the brain. Meanwhile, a thick wad of new questionnaires is ready to be thrown at women, asking about their interest and desire, how lubricated they get during sex and the frequency of their orgasms. As this new wave of measurement breaks around the world, we have to ask how much of it is really in the interests of those being tested, and how much of it is designed to reduce the complexity of women's sexual problems to a simple medical label that can then provide the perfect pathway to a pill.

Not everyone shares the excitement about all the probing taking place out on this new frontier. It's an obsession with measurement some people see as wrong-headed because it's too focused on the genitals and the chemicals. Sometimes medical problems interfere profoundly with the physiological processes of sex—like nerve damage from surgery, for example, which is a situation where a correct diagnosis from a doctor may be extremely valuable. But for Leonore Tiefer and many of her colleagues who work in the sex therapy area and study sexual problems, your sex life is not commonly something you should see a medical doctor about; nor would you get measured to see whether your blood is flowing normally. 'Sex is like dancing,' Tiefer has said. 'You'd see a doctor if you broke your ankle, but not to get tested for your dancing abilities or advice on how to improve your steps.'[3]

Despite the belief that medical technology gives reliable, clear answers, often things are much less certain. A good illustration of the uncertainty is the probe with the unpronounceable name, the photoplethysmograph, which is one way of assessing blood flow in a woman's vagina and is often used in research labs to investigate her level of sexual arousal. The device is essentially a small piece of hard plastic, shaped a little like a tampon and easily inserted by the woman being assessed. Just as with the testing in the darkened room in the medical centre, a woman is shown sexual images or asked to read erotic material, and the high-tech tampon is used to try to measure her responses. Inside there's a tiny light source that shines out against the walls of the woman's vagina. The light measures the way blood pulses through the vagina's walls when a woman is sexually aroused. The measure of the blood's pulsing—technically called 'vaginal pulse amplitude' or VPA—is often used as a way of testing how her sexual response might be affected by an experimental drug.

One of the first problems with using this test is that it's still unclear exactly what vaginal pulse amplitude actually means, even to the sex researchers familiar with its operation who use the test.[4] There is uncertainty about what the pulsing picked up by the little light really represents—whether it may reflect a single process, or a number of different physical processes and events. Complicating matters further, actually reading and understanding the complex results of this test can be difficult, because there may be lots of unwanted material in the computerised data it generates. If, for example, a woman crosses her ankles or tenses her stomach muscles while the test is underway, it can affect the results in ways that are sometimes hard to decipher.

Despite these challenges, VPA has been regarded as an important way to measure women's arousal, and is seen as providing objective evidence of how drugs might enhance it. In a sense, it has become part of the toolkit being used out there on that new frontier of sexual medicine. Its use is not without criticism, however, and some staff at the Kinsey Institute have cautioned specifically against reading too much into the results of this measure. 'Perhaps the most pressing problem,' they say, 'is that researchers know relatively little about precisely what physiologic processes the vaginal photoplethysmograph detects.'[5] While being a useful instrument for research, they argue that the considerable limitations of the test aren't always taken into account. Kinsey Institute research scientist Erick Janssen believes one of the most serious limitations is that it can't be used to compare one woman with the next because it has no scale in the way other measurement tools do. 'It's like using a ruler without marks,' he says. 'We are using this device largely because it is there.' Others have pointed out another obvious difficulty with using the high-tech tampon: putting a small probe into someone's vagina might affect the very processes of her sexual arousal that you're trying to measure.[6]

The attraction of a lot of modern diagnostic technologies, with their flashing screens and complex computer readouts, is that they can give the appearance of providing objective information. The results can be very helpful if you're trying to persuade someone they have a medical condition and need treatment. Sometimes tests can and do provide clear-cut indications of a genuine problem—a different sort of probe can, for instance, help find nerve damage that might have been caused by previous surgery. In such a case, a medical centre might recommend physiotherapy to improve pelvic floor muscles, for example—highlighting the fact drugs are not the only solutions being promoted by doctors and state of the art clinics.[7] But often the results of these diagnostic tests are not so clear cut, and there's a commonly held view that many of the tests—like the high-tech tampon—should not yet be used in routine medical practice.[8]

That still leaves the wider issue that the definitions of the disorders being diagnosed are themselves uncertain, as well as constantly changing. As those Kinsey Institute researchers have pointed out, the 'construct' of women's sexual arousal that the high-tech tampon is supposed to measure remains poorly understood and defined. Likewise, as we'll discover, there is a growing debate about the specific condition known as 'female sexual arousal disorder', another of the disorders of FSD that is becoming increasingly controversial.

There's no implication here that research into the physical side of sexuality is unnecessary, or that shining a light on the walls of a woman's vagina is a joke. Sometimes measurement is entirely appropriate and medical treatment completely necessary. The point is that it might be valuable to ask why doctors are looking so often where that little light is shining, rather than more broadly at all the myriad causes of sexual complaints that lie within cultures, societies, families and relationships. It is always easier to look for your keys in the light of the streetlamp, even though you might have lost them in the darkness around the corner. And the most heavily promoted solutions may be helping to influence the choice of places where we look for the problems.

It isn't hard to realise that researchers may be more interested in measuring women's testosterone because there are drugs that can replace it, scanning female brains because there are pills to affect the levels of its neurotransmitters, and testing blood flow in the vagina because Viagra can improve it. It is important to note that this focus on the physical aspects and the potential of pills comes not just as a result of the emergence of new drugs, but is being driven in part by dissatisfaction among some researchers with the benefits of traditional talking therapies.

In addition, there is a view that many women will want to see the source of their sexual difficulties as physical in nature and may welcome safe and effective medicines as valuable therapies.[9] However, improving genital blood flow alone won't get to the heart of what's causing many women's sexual difficulties. For some women, it might—and identifying them will obviously involve the need for some medical testing. For many others, though, the roots of their dissatisfactions are surely going to be found elsewhere, far from where the light of the high-tech tampon is shining.

As in many other areas of medicine, the understanding of the physical aspects of female sexuality has been influenced by scientific work on animals, including monkeys, dogs and rats. Monkeys are close to humans, but they are hard to keep; dogs are okay, but ethically rats are seen as easiest. One sex researcher has joked that the good thing about rats is that, unlike humans, they don't lie; the problem is that they don't talk either.[10] Rabbits' genitals have also been studied to learn more about women's sexuality. Researchers, including Dr Irwin Goldstein, have used ultrasounds to measure blood flow to the vagina and clitoris of the New Zealand white rabbit in order to understand more about the mechanics of women's sexual arousal. Based on these studies in animals, a team including Dr Goldstein proposed animal models for possible conditions described as 'vaginal engorgement insufficiency' and 'clitoral erectile insufficiency'.[11]

Clearly, there is a view held by many people that work on animals can play a role in advancing scientific understanding about human diseases, notwithstanding the criticisms of animal rights activists. Since at least the early twentieth century, scientists with an interest in sex have been investigating the mating behaviours of animals, in part because, before the work of Kinsey and then

Masters and Johnson, social attitudes meant it was very hard to study the mating behaviour of humans. But for those who see a creeping medicalisation of ordinary life, one impact of all the animal research has been too much focus on the narrow biological aspects of the body, rather than the broader factors at play in human sexuality.[12] Leonore Tiefer has expressed strong doubts about whether animal models of 'engorgement insufficiency' disorders, based on studies of rabbits' genitals, are very helpful in understanding the everyday sexual difficulties of women in Boston or Brisbane. And her doubts reflect a wider question about whether medical doctors are really the best-equipped group within our communities to be dealing with the common sexual problems women face. When asked that question a few years back, the normally urbane Irwin Goldstein quickly turned defensive. 'Who's best equipped to deal with it, the horticulturalists? It's a form of medicine. I think physicians are most appropriate.'[13]

Another of the approaches doctors are using to try to find the source of sexual dysfunction is to measure the amount of testosterone that courses through the female body. Although testosterone is commonly known as the male hormone, women also have it. The view that low testosterone levels cause widespread sexual problems is common among segments of the medical fraternity and the wider public, but it is by no means scientifically proven or universally accepted. Reminiscent of claims that the menopause is a disease of oestrogen deficiency, some have suggested that a testosterone 'deficiency' may cause low desire, which for certain women can then be fixed with help from testosterone drugs. While such an approach may obviously help sell testosterone-based products, it may not necessarily help all the women who take them. Just as with the measures of blood flow and vaginal pulse amplitude, it is not certain what a normal level of testosterone is, and the supposed link between testosterone levels and common sexual problems remains highly uncertain.

'The majority of studies don't find a correlation between testosterone and sexual desire,' a leading Canadian sex researcher concluded after she and her colleagues reviewed the relevant literature.[14] That review of the scientific evidence did not support the belief that a woman's level of testosterone is a key cause of her lack of interest in sex. In fact, the actual levels of testosterone in the body are extremely difficult to measure—there's an enormous variability between different people and levels can change over an individual's lifespan. So deciding on what constitutes a 'normal' reading of testosterone and what level defines a deficiency or dysfunction is proving very challenging. According to that review of the literature, routinely measuring woman's testosterone cannot be recommended as a way of diagnosing sexual problems.

That same review of the evidence casts doubt on that other popular notion: that oestrogen, or the lack of it, is another chief suspect in the sexual whodunit of lost desire. Oestrogen and testosterone are important parts of a bigger group of hormones that do play a role in human sexuality. As a general rule, the levels of these hormones tend to peak and then fall naturally over the length of a person's life, though it is a complex picture. But the scientific evidence does not support making a direct link between changes in the level of one of these single hormones and the bulk of women's common sexual difficulties. There is evidence that falling oestrogen levels after the menopause are associated with difficulties in attaining lubrication, but that doesn't mean all women with low oestrogen levels will experience problems lubricating. There may be cases where very low hormone levels are important factors, but that doesn't mean these levels should be routinely measured in the many women who experience sexual problems. According to the researchers who reviewed the evidence, generally speaking when a woman is 'sufficiently sexually stimulated' the level of oestrogen in her body may well be irrelevant to her capacity for sexual pleasure.

The problem here is not that scientists are interested in studying the physical aspects of sex, the flow of blood or the level of hormones. Their work can produce invaluable knowledge and understanding. The problem is overstating the importance of these physical factors in the wild dance of sexuality, and starting to prematurely measure all manner of things in medical clinics long before we know what the results of all the testing really mean.

Yet undeniably, however important the cultural and historical factors at play, sex does involve a physical act. 'Whatever the poetry and romance of sex, and whatever the moral and social significance of human sexual behaviour,' wrote Alfred Kinsey and his colleagues in 1953, 'sexual responses involve real and material changes in the physiologic functioning of an animal.'[15] While the comments reflect his biologist's focus on the physical, Kinsey was also concerned that the role of hormones and the endocrine organs that produce them was being grossly overplayed, and early versions of hormone replacement over-promoted, even back in 1953:

> Journalist accounts of scientific research . . . [and] . . . over-enthusiastic advertising by some of the drug companies...ha ve led the public to believe that endocrine organs are the glands of personality, and that there is such an exact knowledge of

the way in which they control human behaviour that properly qualified technicians should, at least in the future, be able to control any and all aspects of human sexual behaviour.[16]

Fifty years into the future, the notion that medical technicians and their treatments and technologies can control sexual behaviour is still very much alive. The dream now is that millions of women might be given back their lost desire with a handful of pills, to fix their 'deficiency' of testosterone or the 'insufficiency' of their blood flow. But so far that dream may be more of a pharmaceutical fantasy than a scientific reality.

So, if measuring blood flow or testosterone levels isn't going to unlock the secrets of female sexual pleasure, what about a scan that can look inside a woman's brain, draw back all the curtains of culture and peer at the hard, objective truth beneath? The giant magnetic resonance imaging machines, or MRIs, are in fact being used as another possible means of diagnosing sexual dysfunctions. This time the hunt is on to establish the patterns of brain activity in women with 'normal' sexual arousal, presumably in order to identify the chemical imbalances in women with 'abnormal' arousal, who might then be fixed with drugs. But despite all the colourful pictures these machines can generate—at great expense—MRIs of the brain cannot yet reliably diagnose sexual disorders, or detect how a drug might affect them.[17] As an aside, while the scan of the brain can't yet diagnose sexual problems, it is apparently possible for the machines to visualise what is happening inside a woman's head when she has an orgasm. Apparently the scans can also detect differences between a real orgasm and a fake one, and the more entrepreneurially minded readers may well see another potentially lucrative commercial niche opening up here.[18]

Jokes aside, the medical approach to measuring women's pleasure has confronted genuine obstacles. Even among those who passionately believe in the existence of these sexual disorders in women, there's an acknowledgement that measuring blood flow, testing testosterone levels and scanning brain activity are not reliable ways to diagnose them. So how on earth can doctors discover whether a woman has one of these supposed disorders and needs treatment? And how can drug companies demonstrate that their drugs are working for women if there are no reliable measurement tools available? One answer is the humble questionnaire that can ask women directly how they're thinking and feeling about their sexual experiences.

Questionnaires can be used to diagnose women in doctors' surgeries, or as part of the research process in the trials of drugs or other therapies. But, rather than everyone using the same tool, it seems almost every time a new company wants to start a trial, it wants its own brand-new questionnaire. So, just like the surveys, many of these measurement tools have been developed using industry money—sometimes involving company staff collaborating with outside researchers to actually design them. As we'll discover, in at least one case a drug company has sponsored and helped design the very tool used to diagnose whether a woman might be a candidate for that company's drug.

These questionnaires for measuring pleasure and diagnosing disorders come in all shapes and sizes—long, short, time-consuming and brief. While they appear simple, the science behind them—called psychometrics—is highly sophisticated. In fact, when a senior figure called for the development of a more rigorous science of sexuality back in 1988, he singled out reliable and valid measurement tools like questionnaires as being critical to that project.[19]

To design them, researchers generally start by getting together a list of potential questions, gathered by asking other experts or talking to women in focus groups. Next, a draft set of questions is road tested to see whether they're reliable and do what they're supposed to do. After that, a final set of items is identified and the questionnaire prepared. In some cases, a rating scale is developed to accompany the questionnaire. A woman's answer generates a certain score; the scores are added up at the end of the test; and cut-off points for who's normal and who's not are developed by those designing the scale. If you're above the line you're normal, but if you are below it—bingo! You've got yourself a medical disorder.

Ray Rosen is one of the world's leading authorities on creating questionnaires to measure women's sexual dysfunction, and he's personally worked on designing a number of the new ones that have emerged since the Cape Cod meeting he helped organise back in 1997. Like few others, the charismatic research psychologist understands the science of psychometrics, which can sometimes transform a few answers into the diagnosis of a disorder or show how a drug might have improved things. He's worked on some of the most well-known questionnaires, including the highly regarded Female Sexual Function Index.[20]

Given that it's one of the most widely used tools, and considered one of the best, let's briefly have a closer look at how this particular questionnaire was developed. Luckily it's not too hard to find out how these tools are designed, because it's often all there in black and white in the journal article describing the process. The article on the making of the Female Sexual Function Index was published in 2000, three years after the Cape

Cod meeting, two years out from the launch of Viagra for men and just a year after the famous 43 per cent figure had emerged.[21] As disclosed in the small print of the article, the questionnaire's development was supported at least in part by two drug companies with experimental medicines,[22] which—like Viagra— were believed to enhance blood flow and boost arousal.

So how did Ray Rosen and the team go about developing their questionnaire? They started by asking a panel of experts to nominate potential questions. Next they tried those questions out on a small group of women, to check for basic things like clarity and to see whether they could understand the wording easily. This phase produced a 29-question scale, which then underwent further testing on a larger group of women. After that process, the team then dropped ten items, and finished up with a nineteen-question scale that became the famous Female Sexual Function Index, widely used and still available on the internet a decade later.[23]

The final nineteen-question tool includes items asking how often a woman has felt desire or arousal in the past month, how often she's become wet as part of her sexual activity, how difficult it was for her to reach orgasm, and whether she'd experienced pain during intercourse. But what about the ten questions in the original list that didn't make it into the final version? According to the article describing the process, those ten questions were dropped in order to minimise redundancy and create a briefer instrument. That makes a lot of sense, and things are dropped routinely in the development of these tools, just as they are in any development process. But as an exercise, let's look at which items were dropped; it might shed some light on the way these questionnaires are developed. First, though, a little more background on how these tools are designed and why.

Questionnaires should have what's called in the scientific jargon 'reliability' and 'validity'. Put simply, a reliable tool is one that could be used repeatedly in different situations, but if the same woman filled it out about her experiences, it would give pretty much the same results every time. Validity means that it should measure what it's supposed to measure—in this case, the condition known as female sexual dysfunction.

There are, however, several parts to validity. As Ray Rosen has written, these questionnaires should be able to sort out which women have the dysfunction and which women don't. But crucially, the tools should also be able to detect the effects of treatments, including drugs—or, as Rosen puts it in technical language, the questionnaire needs to be sensitive to 'therapeutically induced change'.[24] In other words, the measurement tool is being designed, at least in part, to be able to detect the effects of drugs and other therapies. The interesting question here is how the underlying reasons for developing a tool affect the way it has been developed.

The interim list of 29 items of the Female Sexual Function Index included a question about the extent to which a woman had 'satisfaction with amount of stimulation from partner', but this question was one of those dropped before the final phase. Why? According to the questionnaire designers, there were three good questions related to the issue of satisfaction already available among the nineteen final questions. This is a perfectly reasonable and legitimate explanation, but one is left with the nagging question about why an item on a woman's satisfaction with the amount of stimulation from her partner would not make it into a final version.

For many involved in the broader debate, like Shere Hite, a lack of adequate stimulation from a partner may be an extremely important cause of much sexual dissatisfaction among women. But obviously it's a factor that it would be very hard for drugs to affect. In other words, if the tool is being designed to help assess the effects of a drug on a woman answering the questionnaire, this particular question may be of little help, because presumably there's not much a drug can do to improve the amount of stimulation a woman will get from her partner. On the other hand, if there's a belief that a drug can enhance lubrication, then questions about how lubricated the woman has become during sex may be more helpful in demonstrating that drug's effect. As it turns out, the final nineteen-item tool includes four questions specifically about lubrication.

Other items dropped from the original 29 items included five questions about how distressed the woman was by her sexual difficulties. Remember that the presence of distress is supposed to be an important part of the medical definition, and without distress a woman doesn't technically qualify for the dysfunction according to the criteria in the *DSM*. Ray Rosen and his colleagues explained that they dropped the questions about distress because of 'ambiguity in their interpretation'. Again, there is no reason to doubt the legitimacy of this explanation. Yet what they then wrote in the next line of their journal article was interesting: 'while distress is an important component in the diagnosis of female sexual dysfunction, the evaluation of pharmaceutical agents will focus on perceptions of sexual responsiveness (e.g. level of arousal and lubrication) and global satisfaction as the clinical outcomes'.

Rosen and his colleagues were reminding us that one of the drivers of the development of this questionnaire was the desire to test pharmaceutical agents. There is nothing wrong with testing drugs before they are widely used—it is a requirement under the law. In fact, the US Food and Drug Administration has explicitly encouraged companies to fund and develop tools to measure the impacts of their drugs.[25] It is fascinating, though, to reflect on how that industry funding may be affecting the way these measurement tools are being developed, and whether in turn these tools might be helping to shape our understanding of the nature of the problem being measured. If you have a ruler, you're interested in length. If you have a thermometer, you're interested in temperature. If you have a drug company-funded questionnaire, isn't it the case that you're more interested in measuring factors likely to be affected by drugs?

Rosen and his team say their tool was designed to assess the 'multidimensional nature' of women's sexual functioning, yet there is clear emphasis on problems of arousal as compared to other problems of desire, orgasm or pain. Almost half of all the questions—eight out of the nineteen items—focus directly on the woman's arousal and lubrication, including the four questions specifically focused on lubrication. The journal article does state that, in the initial phase of developing the questionnaire, an 'emphasis was placed on the selection of items relating to female sexual arousal disorder', though the article offers no clear explanation as to why this emphasis on arousal problems was chosen. Perhaps the emphasis had something to do with the interests of those helping to support the tool's development. One of the companies involved, Zonagen, was at the time testing a drug it believed could enhance arousal and lubrication for women said to have female sexual arousal disorder.[26] Ideally the questions being raised here could have been put directly to Ray Rosen, but he declined repeated requests for an interview for this book.

This industry-supported Female Sexual Function Index is

just one of a series of new measurement tools to have emerged as drug companies have rushed to test their experimental medicines on women all around the world. Soon, a different group of researchers announced they'd developed the Sexual Function Questionnaire.[27] This bigger 34-item questionnaire included items about how often women wanted to have sex, how often they were caressed by their partners as well as questions about arousal and lubrication during sexual activity. This questionnaire was funded by Pfizer at the time the company was hoping its drug Viagra would boost women's arousal. Three of the six authors of the journal article describing the tool's development were Pfizer employees, including the lead author. One of the three non-company employees was Ray Rosen.

Development of this questionnaire had in fact commenced five years earlier, the same year as the historic meeting in Cape Cod that helped to kick start the 'active and positive collaboration' between industry and researchers in this field. That collaboration was certainly beginning to bear fruit. One of the world's leading medical journals had produced 'evidence' that 43 per cent of women suffered from some form of sexual dysfunction and, despite the criticisms of it, high-profile medical clinics were using the figure in their promotional materials. Now scientifically validated tools had been created, and they were ready to measure how drugs or other therapies might improve women's sex lives. The building blocks for this new field of science were quickly falling into place.

A couple of years after the Pfizer-funded questionnaire had been published, the giant P&G was gearing up to start selling its testosterone patch to women. During clinical trials, the company had used questionnaires to measure how its patch was affecting the libido of the women said to have the condition called 'hypoactive sexual desire disorder'. Among the question-naires being used in the trials was yet another new measurement tool, this time the 37-item Profile of Female Sexual Function.[28] The company had funded its development, and the team that developed it had included Procter & Gamble employees.

Part of the reason these questionnaires are worth scruti-nising is that—as with the measures of blood flow, hormone levels or chemical imbalances—they can produce results that look objective and important. They can purport to demonstrate that a drug has dramatically improved a woman's level of desire, attracting the attention of the media and the public generally. Yet on occasions, even if an improvement is 'statistically sig-nificant' it may be of questionable value in the real world of a woman's sex life. A drug may affect the vaginal pulse amplitude of a woman's blood flow, or adjust the mix of neurotransmitters in her brain, without making a scrap of difference to her sexual pleasure or the source of her sexual difficulties. The results of the P&G clinical trials showed that, compared with a placebo or dummy pill, its testosterone patch produced 'statistically sig-nificant' improvements in women's desire, as measured by a scale derived from its own company-funded questionnaire. But the actual magnitude of the improvement over and above the pla-cebo was only six points on a 100-point scale. The meaning of such a small difference for the women involved was 'unknown', according to the health authorities who independently assessed the trial results at the time.[29]

The unreliability of physiological measures like blood flow means that, for many researchers, their scientifically proven questionnaires are the way to go. The changing definitions of the dysfunctions and disorders are no problem, they say, as long as the questionnaires keep adapting. For other observers, these industry-funded questionnaires are focusing too much on measuring the biological aspects of sexual difficulties—like lubrication—because these are the aspects that potentially can be affected by drugs.[30] The broader problem identified by Leonore Tiefer and others is that the measurement tools may be helping to shape—and to narrow—our understanding of what's being measured. No one is blaming the drug companies, though: they're simply taking advantage of an opportunity to help design the tools they need for their trials, with the support and encouragement of government regulators.

With funding from industry, the development of these questionnaires has continued apace, and the trend is towards shorter, quicker tools that are easier to use and can be rolled out across sex clinics and doctors' surgeries all over the world. As the years moved on, Ray Rosen was promoting the idea of simple checklists of questions that could be used to quickly screen patients who might warrant further attention.[31] He maintains that these diagnostic tools are also important to doctors because they can be an 'aid to reimbursement'. If a woman can be classified as having a medical disorder using a scientifically reliable and valid tool, it becomes easier for her doctor to claim reimbursement for the costs involved in her treatment—particularly where there are private insurers involved, as in the United States. So how long should these new screening questionnaires be? According to a presentation Rosen gave at a scientific conference, shorter is better.[32]

If short is beautiful, then the Decreased Sexual Desire Screener is a real stunner. The tool only has five questions and, according to its drug company funders, it can be used by doctors who are not experts in the area to diagnose a woman with FSD in just 'a few minutes'.[33] Though short, this little screening tool could benefit 'millions of women affected by the most common form of female sexual dysfunction, HSDD, which affects nearly one in ten women', claims the company's press release. The German pharmaceutical company that sponsored this questionnaire's development was at the time testing its drug for the very same condition of low desire, 'hypoactive sexual desire disorder', or HSDD.

The first four items of this screening tool ask a woman (1) whether she has had a satisfying level of desire in the past, (2) whether that desire has decreased, (3) whether that decrease is bothersome, and (4) whether she'd like her desire increased. According to the tool developers, if a woman answers yes to these four simple questions, that's enough to provide an 'accurate diagnosis for most patients'.[34] In other words, in the space of a few minutes a woman could be landed with a label that could soon be followed up with a prescription. And all of this might happen without the woman ever knowing that the same folks who would supply the drug to her had helped fund and design the tool being used to help diagnose her.

Unlike some of the other questionnaires, the fifth question in this tool does ask about broader factors at play in the woman's life, like the recent birth of a child, stress or dissatisfaction with a partner. If a woman answering the questionnaire sees any of these things as the source of her 'low desire', it is likely to disqualify her from being diagnosed with a disorder. However, the fine print of the instructions to doctors that accompany the tool leaves the door open to make some sort of diagnosis, even if these other broader factors are at play. The danger is that, in the rushed environment of a short consultation, the complexities of the final question may not be addressed properly. In fact, within a year of its creation, a major company-funded study seemed to be using only the first four questions of the screening tool, rather than the whole five.[35] Notwithstanding this lack of clarity about the role of the fifth question, the purpose of this little screening tool is plain: to allow doctors without expertise in this field to 'identify those women who might benefit from treatment' in just a few short minutes. The researchers who developed the short tool argue that it can be used accurately by non-experts because its ability to diagnose HSDD matches the results obtained by using a longer 'standard diagnostic interview' conducted by experts.[36]

Two of the six researchers who helped create and validate this short screening tool were Boehringer employees. At least one of the drug company employees was involved in every step of the process, from conception and design, through to interpreting data, and then writing and approving the final journal article announcing its validation. The tool designers who were not directly employed by the drug company all had financial ties to it. The lead author of the article on the tool had relationships at that time with more than ten drug companies, including Boehringer—a fact clearly disclosed at the end of the article.

For some researchers, the promotion of tools like the short five-question screener is a cause of great concern. From the perspective of Canadian psychologist Dr Lori Brotto, such tools risk over-simplifying complex sexual problems and giving a woman a label that may not be warranted. She says that in the specialised sex clinic where she works in Vancouver, she might sometimes take up to two hours to make an initial assessment of what's going wrong for a woman and her partner. Brotto, something of a rising star in this field, acknowledges the value of drug companies funding research in an area where it is often hard to get public money. However, she sees the marketing of these 'crude and simple' short questionnaires as an example of the downside of the industry's influence and its unhealthy closeness to researchers.[37] She worries that they are part of a wider push to diagnose disorders too quickly, to identify women with dysfunctions in order to sell them medications. These 'quick and dirty' tools, she says, simply can't investigate all the factors that contribute to a woman's distressing sexual difficulties: 'To quickly make a diagnosis and presume a pill might fix it, we're missing the whole boat here.'

Standing above and beyond this scientific debate about the best way to assess sexual problems—whether with ultrasounds pressed to the clitoris in a darkened room of a clinic or short checklists in the doctor's office—is one of the most sophisticated marketing machines on the planet, currently laying the groundwork for what potentially is a new billion-dollar market among women. As we've seen, the industry's research and development no longer involves just testing drugs; now it includes helping to design the surveys that establish the unmet need for those drugs, and the tools used to decide who needs them. The pharmaceutical companies may not have written the definitions of FSD, but some of them have been trying hard to make sure as many women are diagnosed with the new medical condition as possible. And the next step, another key component of modern pharmaceutical marketing, is funding the 'education' of your local doctor.

Four

Educating doctors with ski trips and strip clubs

Key opinion leaders were salespeople for us, and we would routinely measure the return on our investment, by tracking prescriptions before and after their presentations ... If that speaker didn't make the impact ... you wouldn't invite them back.

—*Award-winning drug company saleswoman Kimberly Elliott*

Sophisticated and stylish, The Mansion on Turtle Creek seems more suited to the realm of fantasy than the reality of downtown Dallas, Texas. Originally the estate of a wealthy cotton baron, the lavish establishment was built in the palatial style of the Italian renaissance. Amidst the soaring arches and giant fireplaces, you can imagine lusty knights and Latin queens engaged in languid conversations and long sessions of illicit lovemaking. Lush, elegant and chic, with lots of intimate space for wining and dining, this world-class restaurant is the perfect location for a romantic liaison. That's why Pfizer chose The Mansion as one of the places at which to 'educate' the good doctors of Dallas about its drugs.[1]

The Mansion is just one of many top-tier restaurants in Texas, and around the world, where the world's biggest drug company has gathered groups of doctors and their dates, plied them with the best food and wine money can buy, and then had them listen to a short presentation from a respected 'key opinion leader'. We've discovered this because one of the company's sales representatives in Texas later became an official government whistleblower. As we'll soon learn, his evidence would join that of other whistleblowers, and inform a massive investigation that left Pfizer facing one of the biggest healthcare fraud settlements in the history of the United States Department of Justice.[2] For its part, the corporation denies almost all the allegations that were made against it in that case, though Pfizer and the government agreed to settle it in order to avoid what they described as the 'delay, expense, inconvenience and uncertainty' of a protracted legal battle.[3]

The facts are that the sumptuous evenings of 'education' at The Mansion and elsewhere were not isolated events. They have been part of a highly effective marketing strategy by one of the most profitable industries on the planet, yet they've remained largely hidden from both patients and the public. When government authorities in Australia tried to urge the global drug giants to reveal details of their wining and dining of Australian doctors, rather than complying with the request for openness drug companies very publicly took a government agency to court. It was a risky gamble, and it failed dismally. The court ruled resoundingly against the industry, and it was forced for the first time anywhere in the world to disclose the details of every single meal it bought for medicos. What the world learned was that, in Australia—which makes up only a tiny fraction of the total global market in prescription medicines—companies were 'educating' doctors at 30 000 events every year, a third of them taking place in restaurants, hotels and resorts, and most of the rest of them in hospitals.[4]

The pharmaceutical industry's tactic has been to blur the lines between promotion and education, targeting the medical profession from the fresh-faced medical students to the greying professors with its sales messages. But, as the world has increasingly become aware, there is no such thing as a free lunch. The scientific evidence on this relationship suggests it can affect the way doctors practise medicine, making them more ready to prescribe all the latest, most expensive drugs.[5] Sometimes a new drug is the most appropriate treatment; however, sometimes a non-drug therapy is better and cheaper, and on occasions simply letting nature take its course is the best strategy of all.

The 'education' of your local doctor starts with the regular visits from the friendly sales reps, helping to arrange the snacks in the surgery, the lunches at the local eateries and the salubrious dinners with influential speakers. The next level up is the company-funded workshops and seminars that happen in universities and hospitals everywhere. After that come the large scientific conferences and big international medical meetings, organised by professional associations whose office staff and scientific journals are kept afloat with the industry's sponsorship. These strategies are commonplace, and this young field of sexual medicine is no different. Behind a doctor's decision to diagnose a sexual disorder lies an extremely tangled web of influence.

In late 1998, a new sales recruit named Blair Collins joined Pfizer, just a few months after the company had launched Viagra for men.[6] Blair was assigned to the Fort Worth district in Texas, to what was then known as Division J. This special sales force was set up to have primary responsibility for selling Viagra, though it sold other drugs as well. Ironically, the initial runaway success of the little blue pill meant there was enormous pressure on sales staff, who were expected to keep increasing sales year by year. In a detailed complaint that would be filed in a court almost a decade later, Blair Collins alleged that over the next few years the company used a long list of promotional strategies to keep those sales growing. Along with the speaker dinners at The Mansion and other favourite nightspots, he alleged there were breakfasts, lunches, coffees, afternoon ice creams and on occasions some very lavish entertainment. Scientists studying the impacts of all this sort of gift-giving stress the importance in human relationships of 'reciprocity'—the fundamental desire to repay a favour that may well be rooted deep in the evolution of our species. For doctors, by and large, the best way to repay a sponsor's favour is by favouring that sponsor's drugs.

According to Collins, doctors were on occasions taken on outings to Broadway-type shows, and offered free trips to high-profile football and baseball games. Pfizer would sometimes pay for a private box at these sporting events, and twenty medicos and their guests would listen to a short presentation before enjoying dinner and the game. There was also an exclusive box at the speedway, where Viagra was a sponsor of the national motor sport, NASCAR, and doctors got to meet the famous drivers. As part of the promotion of a number of other drugs, there was an educational trip to the ski fields in Colorado's Rocky Mountains, as well as excursions to a golf course, a horse race and even a big casino night at a swish hotel, allegations all meticulously detailed in a 194-page complaint filed with the court. And then there was the very special promotional strategy that Blair Collins learnt about on a business trip to Florida: the use of strip clubs.

Still very much the new boy, during an internal company get-together Collins had congratulated one of his more experienced and successful sales colleagues, before asking him how he did it. The way Collins tells it, the colleague indicated that he didn't waste time on the normal methods of marketing drugs to doctors in their offices. Instead, he got together his 25 highest prescribing doctors and took them—two or three at a time—to strip clubs. This isn't the first time drug companies have been accused of using unconventional selling techniques. Just a few years ago, staff members from another pharmaceutical giant were found to have taken a leading specialist to a lap-dancing club in the United Kingdom.[7]

Asked whether he was worried about being fired if his boss at Pfizer knew he was taking doctors to strip clubs, the big shot laughed at the naïve question from the new recruit. He explained that, when he could, the top-selling reps' boss would join them at the clubs. This successful salesperson was not some maverick unknown to his superiors; he was, according to Collins' legal complaint, one of Pfizer's top-selling sales representatives in the United States.

That complaint also alleges that Blair Collins and some of his sales colleagues promoted the idea to influential doctors that Viagra was useful for women, as well as for men, even though it had not yet been approved for that use. So-called 'educational' events about Viagra and women's health were then used to promote that idea more widely. In one case, the sales rep recalled that during the 'question and answer' session following a presentation by an obstetrician and gynaecologist, questions arose about the possible role of Viagra for women. The expert told his audience words to the effect that while the drug was not approved for women, at the university medical centre where he worked they were seeing evidence Viagra could boost women's sexual responses. Collins and his colleagues were then encouraged to hire this same speaker at smaller meetings in their local areas, and to echo those sentiments to as many doctors as they could. After a year or so, when the effects of the initial presentation on prescriptions for women were apparently waning, the same expert was invited back to 'rekindle the embers'.

To keep track of all its educational programs for doctors, Pfizer introduced new software which, according to Collins, allowed management to keep track of which experts were speaking at which meetings. It also encouraged everyone in the company to make sure resources invested in 'education' and other promotional activities were spent as effectively as possible on influential doctors. Another software program was also being used inside Pfizer to keep track of doctors' prescriptions in any given geographical location, over any given time period. When the information gathered from both software programs was used together, Pfizer could allegedly see how its educational programs were affecting prescriptions of its drugs. In the words of Collins' legal complaint, the combination of these two sets of data allowed the company to 'see how effective certain of its programs and/or speakers were in influencing doctors . . . to write prescriptions for Pfizer's drugs'. Put simply, the company was analysing its return on investment in doctors' education.

The lengthy legal complaint filed by Collins' lawyers in the district court alleged that many of these activities were not genuine education, but rather illegal kickbacks and inducements to influence prescribing. In the end, when the case was over, the company would stand accused by US federal and state authorities of having provided kickbacks to doctors as part of the promotion of a total of thirteen of its drugs, including Viagra, though the company strongly denies the allegations.[8] While Pfizer might be the biggest drug company in the world, with parts of its sales forces sometimes apparently pushing beyond the boundaries of the law, this mixing of promotion and education has been standard practice across much of the industry. Over recent years, a small but growing number of whistleblowers like Blair Collins have started to reveal a disturbing picture of what happens inside the many 'educational' events our doctors attend every year.[9] Another member of that small group is Kimberly Elliott.

Since graduating from college in the United States almost two decades ago, Kimberly Elliott has worked almost exclusively for leading drug companies, though not Pfizer. Bright eyed with a winning smile, the saleswoman reaped many awards for her selling along the way, before eventually becoming disillusioned with the industry. After a car accident and a worker's compensation claim, she was fired in 2007 by the company for which she was then working, and decided to part ways with the pharmaceutical industry for good.[10] Part of her job during all those years inside was to develop relationships with top medical experts, otherwise known as 'thought leaders' or 'key opinion leaders'. Within a year of leaving, she'd provided an extremely frank account of the way companies sometimes work with some of these experts. According to Elliott, these men and women were paid more than US$2000 by drug companies for an individual presentation. 'Key opinion leaders were salespeople for us and we would routinely measure the return on our investment, by tracking prescriptions before and after their presentations,' she told the *British Medical Journal* in a plain-talking interview in late 2008, part of which is available on video on the web.[11] 'If that speaker didn't make the impact the company was looking for, you wouldn't invite them back.'

The dinners at The Mansion and others like them are usually organised directly by drug companies, so it's no real surprise marketing executives want to measure the return on investment at these events and see how they affect sales. However, many of the educational events doctors attend are in a different category: they have been sponsored by the industry, but organised more independently by people outside of the companies. These seminars and workshops take place in universities and hospitals year in year out, and are critically important to the way your health professionals think and work, and ultimately the sort of care they offer. Doctors attend them not only because they want to learn about the latest developments in science and medicine to better care for their patients, but because they need the 'continuing medical education' (CME) points these events offer. If a half-day seminar is accredited by a medical association, the doctors who turn up will get a fixed number of points, which goes towards the annual tally they need to keep their professional accreditation up to date.

There are reliable estimates that more than half of all this ongoing education of doctors is funded directly or indirectly by the pharmaceutical and device manufacturers.[12] A lot of the seminars and workshops focus on the nature of diseases, as much as the latest drugs and devices to treat them. The area of 'sexual medicine' is no different. Sponsoring the education of your doctor about female sexual dysfunction—and its sub-disorders—has been part of the strategy of the drug companies, keen to develop markets for their emerging sex drugs. One of those accredited seminars took place in early December

2002, hosted by New York University, around the same time Blair Collins was still busily selling Viagra way down south. For doctors who regularly attend these sorts of seminars, the events that unfolded that Saturday might appear commonplace. But for anyone who hasn't been inside these drug company-sponsored activities, what happened that day will prove a real eye-opener.

Now, let's be crystal clear here: just as Fort Worth, Texas and New York, New York are a long way apart, so too listening to presenters in a large academic auditorium is a world away from strip clubs and kickbacks, and there is no suggestion that sponsors control the curriculum of all CME seminars. On the other hand, it's fairly obvious that educational meetings influence doctors, and sponsors would be unlikely to continue to support seminars where presenters were decidedly unfriendly to their products. Likewise, it is common sense that companies would be more likely to offer financial support to activities where their products might generally be portrayed in a sympathetic light, and the medical need for their use presented as larger rather than smaller.

But is there any hard proof that industry funding does bias doctors' education? There is *not* yet strong scientific evidence proving that funded events are more likely to feature presentations favourable to their sponsors, but there are strong suspicions this is the case.[13] In another recent high-profile court case in the United States, it emerged that industry-sponsored educational events were one of the tools used to illegally promote an epilepsy drug.[14] A report on the topic suggested that with so much CME now sponsored by industry, a pro-drug bias 'has become woven into the very fabric of continuing education'.[15] At this particular 2002 seminar in New York, attended by hundreds of doctors and other health professionals, Pfizer was chief sponsor, the presenters included Pfizer-linked key opinion leaders and Pfizer's Viagra was described at one point as a 'miracle drug'. The auditorium in which the event was held was named the Pfizer Foundation Hall for Humanism in Medicine.[16]

One of the main presenters at the New York seminar was Dr Irwin Goldstein, who spoke about FSD and joined a panel discussion at the end of the day with the other presenters. While others talked about the value of sex therapy, Goldstein was billed to speak about the role of the doctor in dealing with sexual problems. It is important to note that, while the professor of urology and gynaecology works with a medical approach, he acknowledges the multifaceted nature of women's sexual problems, which he believes should be seen within a mind, body and relationships framework.

As an example of his medical approach, with its emphasis on the physiological aspects of sexual problems, at one point in his presentation Dr Goldstein referred to scientific data comparing the testosterone levels of 'normal' women with the levels of his female patients. He told the seminar that on the basis of these data, some women with the dysfunction might have a 'specific defect in steroid synthesis'. This was at a time when Procter & Gamble was still developing its testosterone patch together with a lesser known company called Watson, which happened to be another sponsor of this educational event in New York. There is no suggestion the folks at Watson had any influence over the professor's presentation, but it's not hard to see why they might have been happy with some of his comments. Introducing the idea that some women's sexual problems may be due to a testosterone defect to a room full of many prescribing doctors is obviously going to be beneficial to companies hoping to promote a testosterone fix for that defect. It's also fair to say that the controversy within the scientific literature surrounding the importance of physical factors like testosterone levels, and the broader controversy over the very notion of a widespread condition called FSD, did not come through very strongly during the presentations.

Among the audience members listening from the back of the big auditorium was none other than sex therapist Dr Leonore Tiefer, and one of her colleagues in the New View group, the young sociologist Dr Meika Loe, who had just finished a PhD thesis on Viagra that she was turning into a book. Tiefer happened to be on her home turf at New York University, where she has a position with the department of psychiatry within the medical school. Alarmed by what she saw as a narrow biomedical approach in the program for the drug company-funded educational seminar, she had decided to take the radical step of protesting inside the grounds of her own university. During one of the breaks, the academic activist could be seen distributing leaflets for the recently launched New View campaign. At one point, she even incurred the wrath of one of the urologists attending the seminar, who yelled 'How dare you!' at her across the coffee and biscuits.

'Women's sexual problems and satisfactions have far more to do with relationship difficulties, life stresses, and cultural expectations than with clitoral blood flow or testosterone levels,' argued the inexpensively printed pamphlets, which Tiefer continued to hand out, a little shaken by the abuse but undeterred. 'Don't be misled by drug company-funded marketing masquerading as science or education.' Her campaign was urging doctors to seek their information from non-profit sources, and support more sex education for children and adults. But, rather than education about sex, by the end of the day at the New York seminar the doctors were being educated very directly about sex drugs.

It was after the close of the day's official presentations, and the final panel discussion was about to take place up on stage. But just before the discussion started, as Irwin Goldstein and the other panel members were taking their seats, the panel's chairperson asked the audience to write down any questions they had for the assembled panel members on slips of paper. These were then collected from the audience and passed to the chairperson, who began to pose a series of questions to the panel members. One of those questions was about the idea of men using Viagra on a *daily* basis to prevent sexual problems, rather than every now and again, as was the current recommendation. It appeared to anyone sitting listening to the panel discussion that the question had arisen spontaneously from one of the pieces of paper collected from the large audience.

Rising quickly to the occasion, Irwin Goldstein responded to the chairperson's question about regular use by saying he was a strong believer in men taking the pill on a daily basis to prevent impotence.[17] He told the audience of prescribing doctors and others that he had hundreds of men using Viagra for prevention of sexual problems. 'If you would like to be sexually active in five years' time, take a quarter of a pill a night,' he said with his trademark confidence. 'We have data to show that will facilitate and prolong nocturnal erections.' At that time, the key published evidence to support such a radical endorsement of long-term daily use of Viagra came chiefly from one small study involving 30 men taking the drug for a period of only three nights. Even the folks at the Pfizer headquarters seemed surprised by Dr Goldstein's glowing endorsement of the blue pill. Distancing the company from the comments, a spokesperson said he had not seen convincing data to recommend daily use of the drug to prevent sexual problems.

After the panel discussion had finished, a curious journalist asked the panel's chairperson where the question about daily use of Viagra had come from. The chairperson admitted that he had thrown it in himself, even though it had appeared to the audience as if it had come from their suggestions on the pieces of paper. There's no insinuation Pfizer arranged or influenced the exchange that led to the endorsement of daily use of its drug by a highly respected expert in the field. On the contrary, a company spokesperson appeared genuinely surprised when asked about it. Yet clearly it's the sort of recommendation that could impact very favourably on sales of the sponsor's drugs. It serves as a good example of why drug companies want to sponsor these sorts of seminars, where presenters speak so favourably about sponsors' products. It is also a good reason why it might be worth asking your doctor where they get their education.

On further questioning after the seminar was finished and most of the participants had left the auditorium, the panel chairperson revealed that he'd previously been paid for speaking work by Pfizer. Also asked about his specific links to industry, Dr Goldstein said he'd consulted and lectured for virtually all of the world's pharmaceutical companies—this is, it's important to remember, on top of much of his other publicly funded work. The debonair doctor went on to vigorously reject any concerns about being close to the industry, saying he'd also told the audience at the seminar that Pfizer's drug had a large dropout rate. 'I'm allowed to say what I want,' he told the reporter covering the event. 'No one tells me what to say.' That other independent thinker, Leonore Tiefer, had been watching the whole show. She later described the recommendation that men might take Viagra daily for years as 'bordering on preposterous'. Another leading sex researcher, Dr John Bancroft, called the idea 'scary'.

That seminar in New York was just the beginning. Within a few short years, successive waves of company-sponsored 'education' about FSD, and the drugs to treat it, would be starting to wash across the United States and the world. As with the surveys and the questionnaires, the education was being bankrolled by the pharmaceutical industry in preparation for approval of its new products. Boston University, where Irwin Goldstein was still based at the time, helped develop a package of slides and accompanying notes on male and female sexual dysfunction that would be offered to American hospitals and universities as a half-day accredited education program, supported by an 'unrestricted' grant from Pfizer.[18] The program promised to help give doctors who came along to the seminars practical tips about how to 'expand treatment of sexual dysfunction', according to a letter accompanying the package written by Dr Goldstein. FSD was claimed in the materials to affect up to 63 per cent of women. Yep, that's 63 per cent this time, not 76 per cent and not 43 per cent.

One segment of this particular half-day package was titled 'female sexual circuitry', and it included information about how to understand, diagnose and treat women's common sexual disorders. Along with the psychological, social and cultural causes, problems of blood flow and 'insufficiency syndromes' were singled out. Ultrasounds and vaginal photoplethysmographs— or the high-tech tampon—were also recommended as tests that could potentially provide valuable information. Similarly, doctors were provided with suggestions on how to diagnose women with hormone 'deficiencies'. Questionnaires and scales were also recommended, including the drug company-sponsored Female Sexual Function Index designed by Dr Ray Rosen and his colleagues. One slide was titled 'Identification of FSD', and the accompanying notes stated that while this particular questionnaire had been designed for research purposes, it could be 'useful in clinical practice'. This is despite the fact that the questionnaire's website states directly it was 'not designed for use as a diagnostic instrument'.[19]

In terms of treatment, the half-day CME educational program noted that while no pharmaceuticals had yet been approved for women, drugs including testosterone, despite side-effects and uncertainties about long-term safety, 'appear to help alleviate the dysfunction'. The medicine called sildenafil—the generic name for Pfizer's Viagra—was specifically mentioned in the Pfizer-funded package. One slide boldly stated that the sponsor's drug could improve women's arousal, orgasm and enjoyment, as well as increase the frequency of sexual fantasies and intercourse. These were certainly eye-catching claims, but did not really paint a comprehensive picture of the solid scientific evidence. The notes that came with that slide did add some balance by stating that, while the drug may offer these benefits, trials in older women seemed to show little or no such improvement. Other treatment strategies were also mentioned, including the clitoral vacuum device to increase blood flow and behavioural therapy, described as being highly effective. Psychological approaches and relationship issues were covered in another segment of the educational program, though the overall framework was medical in nature.

Around the same time Pfizer was funding that half-day roadshow, another corporate giant—P&G—was generously sponsoring the education of doctors with another accredited program. Hoping government approval of its testosterone patch might be imminent, the company was funding a short course called Renewing Sexual Desire: Understanding HSDD in Post-menopausal Women. You might remember that HSDD stands for 'hypoactive sexual desire disorder', the disorder of women's low libido P&G was targeting with its testosterone patch.

As it turns out some of the seven educational objectives of the course, clearly stated in its brochure, seemed to coincide with its sponsor's commercial objectives.[20] On completion of the educational activity, the objectives were that doctors should be able to classify the different disorders of FSD, and when it came to treatment they should be able to 'recall the rationale for testosterone use in women with sexual complaints' and 'inter-pret the body of evidence supporting testosterone therapy for the treatment of HSDD'. One doctor who happened to attend the course said she felt like she was 'caught in the middle of a nightmarish infomercial' because it promoted wide usage of testosterone and downplayed its risks.[21] At that time the spon-sor's testosterone patch had not even been approved by health authorities. Two of the three key presenters involved with the course had financial ties to the pharmaceutical industry, with one being a consultant and speaker for four companies, includ-ing the course sponsor. According to the course materials, the chair of the steering committee overseeing the project was Ray Rosen.

Soon drug company-sponsored education about this new dysfunction was going global and moving online. Doctors all over the world could now learn about how to diagnose and treat women at a website called Female Sexual Dysfunction Online.[22] Yet again, the learning was taking place in the long shadows of the drug companies, keen to see the maximum numbers of doctors with pens poised ready to prescribe the moment one of their pills or patches was approved. Sixteen of the twenty educators involved with that online education program had links to the world's major drug companies. One of the editors was again Ray Rosen, who disclosed in the conflict of interest section of the online site that he had consulting or research arrangements with a total of seven drug companies. This whole package of slides and notes—all available free online to doctors keen to help make their annual quota of CME credit points—was supported jointly by 'unrestricted educational grants' from P&G and Boehringer, the German company also hoping to market a drug for the disorder of low desire.

In order to ensure its educational value the online program had undergone a process of 'peer review', according to its website, and it gave the online program a tick of approval. As it happens, the professor who did the peer reviewing disclosed on the website that she had financial ties to four drug firms, including being an adviser to both the companies helping to fund the online package she was reviewing.

More and more, these sorts of financial relationships with drug companies are routinely declared by health professionals. Currently, in most countries, the amount of money flowing into bank accounts as payments for consultancies or advisory work remains a firm secret, though this may change in the near future. Already, in the United States, governments in Vermont and Minnesota require drug companies to report the amounts paid to individual doctors and to make the details publicly available. Pre-empting new national laws, some companies have started to make more information available about exactly what they pay their advisers and consultants within the medical profession. Yet, despite growing disquiet about these relationships, many senior doctors remain unashamed about working closely with the industry and its money, to help try to bring the world new medicines, reliable tools to test those medicines and effective ways to educate doctors about them.

The fact that a company funds an individual seminar doesn't mean its educational value will necessarily be compromised, or that the sponsor has in some way dictated what goes on. Indeed, the doctors and associations that run these sorts of events argue passionately that sponsorship doesn't undermine independence. Sometimes, however, the evidence suggests otherwise. In one case in Australia an educational provider was promoting its seminars to doctors as being 'independent of industry influence', while at the same time offering some sponsors the chance to 'determine a speaker and a topic' for certain presentations, and others the chance to 'work with us to determine a topic that is on message for your product area'.[23]

Confronted with damning evidence from internal company documents and leaked emails, the head of the educational provider said his company had tightened its guidelines for dealing with sponsors, and maintained that all decisions about educational content at his seminars were made independently of sponsor suggestions. He also argued that some level of sponsor involvement in sponsored seminars was standard practice across medicine. Surprisingly, senior pharmaceutical industry figures in both Australia and the United Kingdom have confirmed that the practice of sponsors making suggestions for speakers at sponsored educational events for doctors was not unusual. While many medical professionals are happy with this as the status quo, others see the need for a major clean-up. One recent report called for a comprehensive ban on drug companies sponsoring doctors' education, bluntly noting that 'no amount of strengthening of the "firewall" between commercial entities and the content and processes of continuing education can eliminate the potential for bias'.[24]

Given the commonplace nature of drug company-funded education, it's likely that a good deal of what your doctor has been hearing—or will soon be hearing—about women's sexual problems is happening at seminars sponsored by the companies hoping to sell you drugs—unless, of course, your doctor is one of those who's stopped accepting the free lunches and no longer goes to the sponsored CME. The idea that women's sexual complaints are the symptoms of disorders and dysfunctions that are widespread and treatable is central to much of this company-funded education. Yet that is just one controversial perspective within a broad-ranging global debate over how to understand women's sexual difficulties, and how to deal with them. Though her perspective has often been left out of these industry-sponsored educational activities, Leonore Tiefer's voice is gaining increasing legitimacy and attention. The campaign she kicked off has moved up in the world since she was distributing leaflets that day in December back outside the Pfizer auditorium. The New View approach to women's sexual problems has its own teaching manual, an accredited CME package available via the internet and its own meetings, though it doesn't have quite the firepower of the pharmaceutical industry to help promote it.

Sponsored seminars are simply more strands in the tangled web that link doctors and pharma companies in a million different ways, with potential effects on how our health problems are understood and treated. It's not just the intimate dinners at posh restaurants and educational seminars at university lecture halls that are being funded. It's also the giant international scientific meetings of experts that happen regularly in swish hotels all over the world, like the one about women's sexuality that took place in Atlanta, Georgia back in the autumn of 2004.

In late October in this southern city there's still a sensual steaminess in the air, and after dark a soft haze wraps itself around the pools of light lining the streets. Like a lot of other centres across the nation, Atlanta has been something of a corporate town, home to Coca-Cola and the 24 news channel CNN. It was also the setting for one of Tom Wolfe's searing critiques of the business of American life. Just like the food industry and the media, in health care it's the giant corporate conglomerates that wield the real power. As the conference participants arrived at the Atlanta Hyatt Regency, streaming past the potted palms and blue-suited African-American porters, the first thing they saw as they lined up to register was the prominently displayed sign offering 'sincere appreciation' to the major corporate sponsor of this scientific gathering, Pfizer Inc. A second sign not far away noted 'special thanks' to all six of the corporate sponsors. Five were drug makers, including P&G. The group holding the meeting in Atlanta was the International Society for the Study of Women's Sexual Health, created largely through the energy and enthusiasm of Dr Irwin Goldstein a few years earlier. Unlike some of the other groups of sex researchers, such as the International Academy of Sex Research, this new organisation happily relies on sponsorship from drug companies, whose staff mingle with participants in the coffee breaks and take their seats inside the lecture theatres during the scientific sessions.

In addition to the industry funds supporting the conference, almost one-third of all the speakers at the Atlanta meeting disclosed that they had financial relationships with drug companies.[25] The relationships ranged from working on company-funded clinical trials to holding stocks and shares.

Many of the researchers who disclosed they had financial ties were paid speakers, consultants or advisers to drug companies, while at the same time holding down senior positions at universities. A dozen of the presenters, including some of the most influential researchers in the world in this field, declared they had ties to three or more drug companies. A high-profile British researcher scheduled to give one of the keynote addresses at the Atlanta meeting, Dr John Dean, revealed he had relationships with no less than eleven companies. The chairperson of the entire scientific program for the meeting was Dr Anita Clayton, who matched John Dean with her own ties to eleven different drug and device companies.

These may seem extraordinary levels of conflicts of interest to those looking on from outside medicine, but it is important to note this is not a case of those paying the piper calling the tune. The doctors and the drug company staff mingling among the pot plants develop connections born from their common goal of treating what they believe to be a massive unmet need among women. And despite the many financial relationships between drug companies and those responsible for developing and delivering the scientific program, the Atlanta meeting boasted many presentations that had nothing to do with drugs. Along with genital blood flow and testosterone, speakers touched on everything from the damaging role of childhood abuse to the devastating problems of pain with intercourse and the potential sexual benefits of chocolate. Similarly, the presentations by key opinion leaders linked with the drug industry often emphasised the critical role played by personal relationship issues in women's sexual problems—an approach that doesn't help the companies promoting drug solutions.

For those wondering about the sexual benefits of chocolate,

the results presented in Atlanta were, sadly, not that promising. A group of Italian researchers had asked 150 women to complete a battery of sex questionnaires and also answer questions about their chocolate intake. Although there was a faint association between having a positive attitude to chocolate and getting higher scores on sex questionnaires, there was no real evidence chocolate helped women's sex lives—though, as they always say, more research surely is necessary.[26] Perhaps Lindt might even fund it?

The sponsors' role at all these events is not normally in the form of ham-fisted clumsy manipulation, whether they are small educational gatherings in Manhattan or Melbourne, or large scientific meetings in Atlanta or Paris with hundreds or even thousands of participants. The flow of influence is much more subtle and far more profound. The pharmaceutical industry, like a modern God of Science, is omnipresent in the lives of many doctors, with friendly marketing folk popping up almost every time a group of health professionals meets for a drink or a chat, whether it's a hotel lobby, a medical centre's lunch room or an up-market strip club. For companies, the big scientific meetings are the perfect opportunity for staff to mix freely with prescribing doctors and rub shoulders with the leading experts at the peak of their power and influence, while also starting to cultivate the next generation of key opinion leaders.[27] Yet the flow of influence is not always so subtle. As former drug salesperson Blair Collins explained it, from the industry's point of view, the primary aim is always expanding markets for medicines. Pfizer's mode of operation was to develop relationships with 'key opinion leaders' and then use those doctors 'to help sell the drug to other doctors and to train other doctors to sell the drug. These key opinion leaders were recruited through educational grants (restricted and unrestricted) and other incentives and by the promise of future lucrative speaking engagements.'

As part of the research for this book an interview was requested with Pfizer, and among the long list of topics flagged for discussion was its historic settlement with the United States Department of Justice, of which Blair Collins' complaint was part. The company chose to decline the offer of an interview but instead sent a response that made no mention of the settlement or the allegations against it as part of that case.[28] The response did, however, state that Pfizer had conducted or sponsored many studies in the area of FSD including surveys, questionnaire development and drug trials, but that it had not conducted any 'disease awareness' campaigns for the condition. The response also included a general comment on Pfizer's funding of educational activities such as the Atlanta conference, its relationships with health professionals and partnerships with organisations:

> Pfizer partners with many medical, scientific, patient and civic organizations to support their programs and activities, such as health education and scientific research. This support takes many forms, including grants and charitable contributions for efforts that strengthen communities, and work toward a healthier world. Working with these organizations allows Pfizer to better understand the needs of the patients who take our medicines, while helping these medical, scientific and patient organizations inform and address the needs of those they serve.

Scientific meetings like the one in Atlanta are also the perfect forum to release important new information about a sponsor's latest products, in an environment where there is some—albeit a limited—degree of influence. If the sponsor plays its cards right, it can generate lots of enthusiastic stories in the media too, helping create a positive buzz about its soon to be released blockbuster. The Atlanta meeting was taking place just a matter of weeks before a critical assessment of the testosterone patch by the US Food and Drug Administration. The forthcoming public hearings would be the first-ever such assessment of a drug for female sexual dysfunction. So, as a sponsor of the Atlanta meeting, P&G took the opportunity of giving the gathering of sex researchers—and the world—a sneak preview of the latest scientific data about its new testosterone patch for women.

Company employees were part of the team that had run the studies of the company's drug and they presented up-beat results from those studies at a meeting where that same company was one of the sponsors. The buzz about a possible forthcoming drug approval was in fact something of a feature of the scientific gathering in Atlanta, with one speaker proclaiming excitedly that the world of sex research was poised at an important moment in history. When the complete data from the company trials were publicly analysed at the independent regulators hearings a few months later, however, a rather less flattering picture of the testosterone patch would emerge.

That sex conference in steamy Atlanta was also significant because it marked another milestone in the development of this new field of sexual medicine. The first-ever issue of the newly created *Journal of Sexual Medicine* had come out just a few months before, and it was enthusiastically distributed at the conference complete with a glossy full-page blue and white advertisement as its back cover: 'Viagra: powerful performance when you want it.' Such is the norm, as many medical journals rely heavily on drug company advertisements to fund them. As it happens, despite the glossy back cover featuring Pfizer's ads, this new journal is relatively free of advertising compared with most.

The *Journal of Sexual Medicine* would quickly become a place where much of the emerging science of FSD would be published, including studies funded by industry. It wasn't just the researchers getting their articles in print who were celebrating. Drug company executives welcomed the new journal so effusively that the journal's editors decided to note the industry's endorsements on the journal website.[29] Of two endorsements on the website in 2009, both came not from independent doctors or professional associations, but rather from drug company employees. A Pfizer guy endorsed the journal as the 'preeminent, peer-reviewed source' for the science of sexual function and dysfunction. An executive from another drug company described it as the 'journal of choice' in the field. The journal's editor-in-chief was the tireless Dr Irwin Goldstein, and its editorial assistant was his wife, Sue Goldstein, who would mention in an impassioned editorial a few years later that she had sought and received treatment for female sexual dysfunction.[30] Both Irwin and Sue Goldstein declined requests to be interviewed for this book.

Very quickly the *Journal of Sexual Medicine* has grown in stature, as demonstrated by its rising 'impact factor', one of the key measures of success used in the world of medical journals. A journal's 'impact factor' comes in the form of a simple number, and is derived from how often articles from that journal are cited in other articles—including articles from the same journal. This practice is called 'self-citation'. As the editor of the *Archives of Sexual Behavior*, a competing journal, has unkindly pointed out, the new *Journal of Sexual Medicine* has an impressive 'impact factor', but it also has a very high rate of self-citation. 'For the narcissistically inclined, "Self Citations" is not a bad way to be noticed,' wrote the editor, starting a minor skirmish in the world of sex journals.[31]

An associate editor of the *Journal of Sexual Medicine* hit back quickly, defending the high rate of self-citation in his journal and rejecting any suggestion that there was a policy encouraging self-citation among authors. He also revealed that his journal's already high rate of self-citation was going up, not down. He noted that over 50 per cent of the references to articles in the *Journal of Sexual Medicine* actually came from other articles in the same journal. This is in fact a rate of self-citation many times higher than that of some of its competitor journals. The reasons, he speculated, were that his new journal had quickly become a 'flagship' for the field, and the material it published was highly important.[32]

Perhaps just a symptom of healthy competition between medical journals, this petty conflict also helps to show the rough and tumble out on the frontier of this new field of medical science. The creation of the new *Journal of Sexual Medicine* is certainly another pillar in the temple of the science of sexual disorders. It's also become the official journal of the International Society for Sexual Medicine, or ISSM, another professional association happy to accept industry sponsorship of its activities. One of the presidents of that esteemed global society has been British general practitioner Dr John Dean, the man who's had more financial ties to drug companies than you can poke a stick at.

A big friendly Englishman, John Dean has been trying to delicately walk a very fine line. He's one of the captains of the new ship of sexual medicine, acutely aware that drug company money has been keeping the whole show afloat: the research, the surveys, the questionnaires, the conferences, the international societies and the education of doctors. Despite his positive outlook and affable air, Dr Dean can also see the dark clouds of public concern about doctors' cosiness with the pharmaceutical industry looming on the horizon. 'We have buried our heads in the sand a little bit over this over the years,' he said during a long and very candid interview.[33] 'There are important issues here that we have neglected; perhaps we are a little too cosy; a little too comfortable.'

In the small world of sex research, John Dean had happened to find himself on a formal committee with Leonore Tiefer, examining ethical issues like how to manage the financial relationships between doctors and drug companies. Like a lot of people, he was familiar with her criticisms of, and concerns about, companies becoming so intimately involved in building the science of women's sexual dysfunction. Where some proudly see industry's role as paramount and the collaboration with it as positive, Tiefer sees it as fundamentally distorting. She doesn't even regard 'sexual medicine' as an established clinical sub-specialty at all. Rather, she says, 'sexual medicine' is 'the brand-name for a product being aggressively promoted by a multi-billion dollar industry'.[34] Asked whether he believed there was a danger the agenda and work of his international association and its influential members could be distorted by the closeness with drug companies, Dean was clear: 'I think that I would accept that there is a significant risk of that. We need to develop a strategy in the future, so that we can reduce the risk of the agenda being distorted.'

Dean argued that what are referred to as 'private–public partnerships' between the corporate sector and public institutions are being actively encouraged at the highest level of government in many nations, and that doctor–drug company connections are another positive example of those partnerships at work. Moreover, doctors and drug companies have something of a shared agenda anyway: to get safe and effective medicines to people who need them. But, as he's also acutely aware, that agenda is not—and can never really be—the same. For industry, its duty to shareholders means maximising the numbers of people portrayed as needing their drugs, and FSD has been regarded as a billion dollar market waiting to happen. For doctors, the duty and motivation are supposed to be entirely different.

For John Dean, despite his multiple ties to companies hoping to sell drugs to women, his years as a family physician have produced a deep understanding of the role that relationships and life circumstances can play in causing sexual difficulties. For him, all that experience puts the need for pills into a proper context. 'Drugs are a small part of the care of people with sexual problems. For the majority of sexual problems, drugs really have very little role to play,' he said. Pushed to explain what medical education might look like in an ideal world, he said that in his view doctors' learning could be funded through entirely independent sources, without drug company money. As we'll learn, that ideal may be closer than many people think, as the global push for genuinely independent education of our doctors and other health professionals gathers steam.

Not long after Dean's interview, the world discovered that Pfizer, one of the sponsors of his group's activities, had been involved in one of the biggest cases of healthcare fraud in United States history.[35] At the centre of the case were allegations that a Pfizer subsidiary had illegally promoted an anti-arthritis drug for conditions for which it was not approved, creating safety risks to the many patients being targeted. Admitting to certain limited guilt surrounding those allegations, Pfizer agreed to pay the government US$1.2 billion, the biggest criminal fine in the history of criminal prosecution in the United States. According to the government's fact sheet on the historic settlement, the drug company used 'so-called advisory boards, consultant meetings and other forums and remuneration, including travel to lavish resorts' to illegally promote its drug to doctors. It also sponsored 'purportedly independent continuing medical education programs' to help promote unapproved uses of the anti-arthritis drug. In some ways, the blurring of promotion and education was at the heart of the fraud.

On top of the billion dollar plus criminal fine, Pfizer also had to pay out US$1 billion dollars in civil penalties. This was in connection to a range of allegations, including that it had paid kickbacks to doctors to promote thirteen of its drugs, including Viagra, as had been alleged so eloquently in the legal complaint made by Blair Collins, the former sales rep turned whistleblower. Under the terms of the final settlement, Pfizer continued to maintain a blanket denial of virtually all the specific allegations against it, though at the same time the government prosecutors continued to assert that their claims were well founded. Both sides eventually agreed to settle, with the fines and associated penalties totalling US$2.3 billion, in order to prevent an even longer legal case.

Importantly, despite the unprecedented size of the criminal fine, under the settlement between the government and the giant company not one individual executive faced a jail term. This fact did not go unnoticed by the sentencing judge, who expressed his concern that there was a strong sense of incompleteness in the criminal case involving Pharmacia—the company acquired later by Pfizer.[36] 'This is a case in which no human being, apparently, is going to be held responsible for substantial criminal activity by a corporation,' said district court judge Douglas Woodlock in his sentencing remarks. He went on: 'It has, I think, become something of [a] cost of doing business, a very high cost of doing business, for some of these corporations to shed their skin like certain animals and leave the skin behind and move on to the future without ultimately giving the public what it is entitled to, which is the satisfaction of knowing that there has been full evaluation of the criminal responsibility of the individuals who occupied that skin.'

Describing these caustic comments as merely his personal reservations, the judge said he accepted the terms of the settlement, which he felt were 'fair and reasonable'. He also expressed the hope that things might change within the world's biggest drug company, because as part of settlement there was a new 'corporate integrity agreement' with the government. Around the same time a Pfizer spokesperson was quoted as saying: 'We regret certain actions taken in the past, but are proud of the action we've taken to strengthen our internal controls and pioneer new procedures.'[37]

As part of that 2009 agreement, Pfizer made commitments to be more open about its marketing behaviour, and agreed to be monitored by external reviewers. Yet here was history repeating itself in the most blatant way. It had only been seven years previously, back in 2002, that the same company had made similar commitments to clean up its act with more openness, and signed a previous 'corporate integrity agreement' with government following an earlier hefty fine.

As part of that earlier integrity agreement, Pfizer introduced what it termed an 'open door' policy within the company. The policy encouraged any staff member who witnessed illegal conduct to come forward, and promised them protection from retaliation. It was in fact this very policy that encouraged a Texas sales representative called Blair Collins to report a number of concerns to Pfizer management in 2003. But, rather than protection, Collins got retaliation and was ultimately terminated. Years later, though, his meticulously documented allegations would contribute to the much bigger case against the company, settled finally with those historic fines. By law, whistleblowers can qualify to receive a portion of fines paid by corporations as a result of their testimony. Being one of the official whistleblowers, Blair Collins received over two million dollars for his troubles.

Meanwhile, as the billion-dollar settlement was being signed, the little blue pill Collins had started selling soon after it came on to the market was about to celebrate its twelfth birthday.

Five

Viagra turns twelve

At first I thought it was great but now I'm worried that . . . he might be getting reliant on it . . . and in some ways, you know, I don't even like thinking about that, cause it's like 'God, does someone have to take a pill to have sex with me?'

—33-year-old woman whose partner took Viagra

Single and well educated, the fit 40-something male works in the media and lives in a large Canadian city. He has also used Viagra recreationally, and he now regularly obtains prescriptions for Cialis from his doctor. 'I was scared shitless the first time I ordered it,' he revealed candidly, agreeing to an interview on the condition he remained anonymous. 'I was trying to convince my doctor that I wasn't impotent.' Frequently exposed to Viagra ads in nightclub washrooms, our anonymous man says his decision to first try the drugs was not driven by the marketing. Asked about the factors influencing his decision to switch pills, he said he read a magazine article in which women's testimonials about great sexual experiences mentioned that their partners were using Cialis.

If you want to peer into the future of how the condition called female sexual dysfunction might play out, it will help to take a look at what's happened with erectile dysfunction and the new sex drugs for men. Initially marketed to an older, more defined group of men with physical problems such as diabetes or prostate cancer, the blue pill and its competitors were soon being promoted as something that might help almost every man, generating combined sales of billions of dollars a year. Three key steps have helped to bolster those sales enormously: redefining erection problems as the sign of a medical dysfunction, widening the numbers said to be affected as much as possible, and then selling a drug as a simple fail-proof solution.

It was back at a major publicly funded conference in 1992 that the new medical term 'erectile dysfunction' came to prominence, six years before Viagra would hit the market.[1] Unlike the ugly word 'impotence' that it replaced, erectile dysfunction was more clinical, more physical, making no judgement about the man's potency. But it also implied the problem was that a man's penis wasn't functioning properly. His feelings and relationships were in a sense left out of the picture. Huge claims of how many men suffered from erection problems soon helped to firm up this new approach, framing them more as medical symptoms outside of the relationship contexts in which they occurred. One high-profile survey claimed that over half of all men over 40 had some kind of erection problem.[2] As we'll discover, that big statistic was only possible because any problem a man had obtaining an erection, even if it was minimal, was added into the totals. And to help show that these problems could affect anyone—no matter how manly and athletic—the pharmaceutical industry hired sports celebrities all over the world to urge men to talk to their doctors about this common, under-treated 'condition'. There were baseball stars in the United States, hockey stars in Canada and soccer stars in Latin America and Europe—all paid handsomely to help promote a similar message: a solution was now at hand.

Viagra works to help men have erections by harnessing a chemical called nitric oxide that causes blood vessels to relax, thereby increasing the flow of blood to the penis. It was the first pill that effectively improved a man's ability to obtain or maintain an erection, making it much easier to use and a lot more palatable than earlier alternatives involving vacuum pumps or injections into the penis.

It's certainly the case that, for some men with physical problems that cause erection problems, these new drugs can be effective treatments. When Viagra was first launched, older couples were used as models in advertising, and the United States ex-presidential candidate Bob Dole appeared in Pfizer's commercials, speaking about his experiences using the drug after he'd had surgery for prostate cancer.[3] Messages like this have rightly been credited with helping to de-stigmatise erection problems and allowing men to speak about what was a source of hidden personal shame. But as those who've tracked the advertising have observed, within a few short years the marketing strategy was shifting from a focus on older men and men with medical problems to a much broader and younger age group.[4] In the United States, one of the few places in the world where it is legal to promote prescription pills direct to the public, there have been some classic advertisements helping to broaden the drug's reach.

One magazine ad featured a close-up photo of a ruggedly handsome man around the age of 40 with the bold headline: 'Viagra. It works for older guys. Younger guys. Even sceptical guys.'[5] Then, in the small print, the ad asked its readers: 'Think you're too young for Viagra? Do you figure, "It only happens once in a while so I'll live with it"? Then nothing's going to change, especially your sex life.' The message was clear: even the most occasional erection problems could benefit from being treated with a drug. It wasn't long, though, before the marketing seemed to be reaching out to an even wider group—men like our anonymous Canadian who weren't impotent at all, but simply wanted to enhance their sex lives. For North American readers a lot of this advertising will be all too familiar, but for people living elsewhere the audacity of some of the claims will be simply fascinating.

One high-profile television commercial featured a man and a woman walking down the street, shopping. They first look at high-heeled shoes and the man then admires a mannequin in sexy black underwear, as the voice-over says: 'Remember that guy who used to be called "Wild Thing?" The guy who wanted to spend the entire honeymoon indoors? Remember the one who couldn't resist a little mischief? Yeah, that guy.' At this point, Viagra-blue horns sprout from behind the man's head to a blast of trumpet. 'He's back,' says the ad triumphantly, as the horns then become the V for Viagra.

And pretty soon Pfizer wasn't the only company doing it, as the industry brought us Levitra and then later Cialis, with their rounds of promotion helping to further expand the market. Amid images of a woman's flashbacks to romantic moments, a television commercial's voice-over asked: 'In the mood for something different? How about Levitra? Ask your doctor if Levitra is right for you. It's the best way to experience that difference.' The approach must have worked. For this class of medicines, the drug companies were soon spending far more on these advertisements than they were spending on sending sales representatives to visit doctors.[6] Normally, it's the other way round.[7]

This focus on advertising to the public as a key promotional tool is very closely linked to how the condition of erectile dysfunction, or ED, has been expanded far beyond earlier definitions of male impotence. Inflated estimates of how many men suffer from the condition have subtly been mixed with suggestions that any degree of inability to have an erection, at any time, is too much. The implied message from so much of the advertising is that a younger man's sexuality is the norm against which all men, at any age, should measure themselves. And that means the changes in sexuality that happen as we age can become portrayed as medical problems to be treated. That a man may have grown in experience and sensitivity as he's aged, and may have become a better lover as a result, is simply not part of the picture. This construction of new norms is certainly something for which to watch out as the campaign to promote female sex drugs intensifies.

A New York urologist who'd been a speaker for Pfizer was quoted in a book about Viagra saying just about every man over 50 could use a little fixing: 'People think that they have to have severe ED to take Viagra. But that's not true. It works well for men who can get erections, but the erections aren't as rigid as they once were. Or they don't last as long as they used to. Or there may be a longer interval between erections. Now, I prescribe Viagra for men of all ages. But I think just about every sexually active man over 50 could benefit from Viagra.'[8] A similar viewpoint came from an executive at Bayer, one of the drug companies that markets Levitra. 'It's going to be important to communicate to men that it's okay,' she said. Erectile dysfunction is 'just a natural consequence of aging. Kind of like when you reach the age of 40 and you start to need eyeglasses.'[9]

In countries that ban the advertising of prescription drugs on television and in magazines, there's nothing to stop drug companies running campaigns to raise public awareness about the conditions their drugs will target. In Australia, soon after Viagra was launched, Pfizer was funding huge advertisements in leading newspapers, promoting the idea erection problems were widespread and that they were the symptoms of a treatable medical condition. 'Some people think erection problems are just a normal part of ageing, so there's nothing you can do about it. That's simply not true. It's a medical condition,' the Pfizer advertisement said. 'Restore your sex life. Talk to your doctor today.'[10] Another advertisement—this time a full double-page spread—claimed that almost 40 per cent of men who visited doctors had erection problems, echoing the statistic about half of all men over 40.[11] As with the famous 43 per cent statistic for FSD, these large figures paint a distorted and misleading picture.

The 40 per cent figure used in the Australian advertising comes from a study that added together all men who had erection problems 'occasionally', 'often' and 'all the time'.[12] The proportion of the men in that study who were aged in their forties who had problems 'all the time' was actually only 2 per cent, while for men in their seventies it was closer to 50 per cent. Other studies around the world suggest rates of erection problems much lower than the 'over half of all men over 40' claim that has attracted much attention. A huge Swedish survey in the city of Gothenburg found that fewer than 10 per cent of men over the age of 45 reported they had impotence.[13] When those figures are broken down by how old the man was, the problem is put more into perspective. The rates of impotence among men aged 45 to 50 were less than 2 per cent. For men aged 80 to 85, the figure was 18 per cent. A review of several different studies reported that between 3 and 9 per cent of men have difficulties with erections.[14]

So what is the basis for the claim that over half of all men aged over 40 have erectile problems? One key source is the Massachusetts Male Aging Study.[15] This was a study of just over 1700 men living in the area around Boston in the late 1980s, and Dr Irwin Goldstein was one of its chief investigators. The headline finding from the survey was that 52 per cent of men aged between 40 and 70 had some degree of impotence. The methods used in this study were a little complicated and, as others have observed, there are caveats that should accompany the dramatic headline result.[16]

One key complication was that the study involved two groups of men: a larger initial group and a different smaller group of men surveyed a couple of years later. Only those in the smaller group were asked to rate themselves as to how impotent they thought they were: not at all, minimal, moderate or completely impotent. The researchers hadn't asked the initial larger group that specific question—at least in part because, at the time this survey started, the understanding and assessment of erection problems was undergoing major changes. Using complex statistical processes, the answers from the smaller group were then used to estimate what the answers would have been from the initial larger group of men had they been asked the same question. In this way the researchers came up with the totals of 52 per cent, though if you remove the men estimated to have 'minimal' impotence the figure dropped down to 35 per cent. The reliability of this 35 per cent figure is also questionable, though, because the evidence from a follow-up survey a few years later suggested it was likely to be an over-estimate of the true extent of these problems.

That later follow-up study was conducted by some of the same researchers and published almost a decade later. As part of that follow-up, almost all of the original survey participants were directly asked about the degree to which they considered themselves to be impotent. One of the interesting results was that, out of 125 men originally classified as completely impotent, 63—or half—were reclassified as not at all impotent.[17] Overall, the results of the follow-up study suggested the total number of men with any sort of erection problem was 44 per cent, not 52 per cent. This time around, if you removed those men classified as having 'minimal' erectile dysfunction, the overall rate dropped to around 20 per cent.

Despite the fact that the headline figure of 52 per cent from the original study gives an exaggerated sense of the problem, it continues to be cited. An erectile dysfunction website in the United Kingdom, for example, states that 'as many as 1 in 2' men over 40 suffer from erectile difficulties, referencing the original Massachusetts study as the source of the evidence rather than the later follow-up which had the lesser estimates.[18] That website was funded by Bayer, which says its figures are in line with other research in the area, and is just one of many company-funded sites trying to educate the world about the very condition their drugs are targeting. A study of websites about erectile dysfunction found company sites were often the first that popped up on an internet search of the term, and were usually within the top two or three sites.[19]

One website in Canada features a large cartoon elephant sitting in the bed between a disgruntled looking man and woman, with the tag line at the bottom of the page saying 'take me somewhere else'.[20] The website claims that 'up to 95% of ED cases are treatable'. Nowhere on the website is there any suggestion

that sexual problems might be treated through talking therapies; only drugs and devices are mentioned. Without saying it
outright, the statement suggests 95 per cent of men who suffer
from erection problems can take a medicine and have their problems solved—which does not match up with the facts. Certainly
these drugs are effective, as we'll see, but not that effective. The
website also includes a quick five-question online quiz called
the 'ED test', where if a man admits to the slightest difficulty
he's told his ED severity is 'mild' and he should speak with his
doctor. It's hard to tell from a quick visit, but the small print in
the 'terms and conditions' reveals the Canadian site is funded
directly by the manufacturer of Cialis, Lilly, whose drug is subtly highlighted in the information provided.

Arguably such a website violates national laws in Canada that
prohibit direct-to-consumer advertising of prescription medicines. It also potentially violates international ethical criteria for
drug promotion, which condemn disguised promotion.[21] These
criteria, produced by the World Health Organization, are not
legally binding. Many national governments prohibit misleading or deceptive advertising, but tend to turn a blind eye to
company-sponsored websites that don't include direct advertising for a specific named brand, even if they seem very obviously
promotional. This site—along with many like it—is especially
telling for what it omits. The only reference to relationships is
the cartoon image of the disgruntled couple representing the
'pre-treatment' situation and another cartoon of a happy couple,
presumably 'post-treatment'. Erection difficulties are constructed
as a cause of relationship problems that can be solved with a
drug, or other medical interventions. The idea that relationship
difficulties, emotional or life problems can contribute to sexual
difficulties is seemingly absent.

In response to a series of questions, Lilly's Canada office said its website aimed to educate men over 40 and their partners about erectile dysfunction.[22] The company statement claimed the condition affected more than 30 per cent of Canadian men, and that 80 per cent of cases may be due to a physical cause. Asked specific questions about whether its site violated national laws and WHO guidelines, and whether its promotion was pitched at men with mild problems, the company statement failed to respond directly, stating that the website had been reviewed by the self-regulatory body, Advertising Standards of Canada.

This notion that men's sexual problems can be solved through the quick fix of a pill is underpinned in some ways by social stereotypes about male sexuality and potency—stereotypes sometimes reinforced on drug company websites designed for the public. Two researchers, Cecilia Åsberg and Ericka Johnson, have analysed the way masculinity was presented on Pfizer's website in Sweden, and they've described what they call the construction of 'Swedish Viagra man'.[23] According to the two researchers, before developing its website the American drug giant hired a polling company to find out what qualities Swedes associated with manliness. The top ten qualities identified in Pfizer's poll, in order of frequency, are outlined in the box.

Top ten qualities of Swedish men according to Pfizer's poll

1. Being practical and able to fix things
2. Potency
3. A well-paying job
4. An attractive partner
5. A physically fit, muscular body
6. Attractive appearance

---

7. Interest in sports
8. Always being ready for sex
9. Owning technical gadgets
10. Having a cool car

It's hard to miss both the stereotypical representation of male roles in this list and the embedded links to Pfizer's product, particularly the ideas that to be masculine is quintessentially to have 'potency' and always be 'ready for sex'. The company's Swedish website on male potency ultimately did not name Viagra, consistent with national laws that prohibit advertising medicines to the public. The website was, however, coloured Viagra-blue and featured a picture of a man in Viagra-blue overalls changing a tyre on a Viagra-blue car. The site also tapped extensively into national imagery of the rugged outdoor life as a symbol of masculinity. 'Viagra,' the researchers observed, 're-aligns the man to his natural virility.'

Apart from helping to reinforce certain versions of masculinity, the promotion of the new drugs has meant that the term 'erectile dysfunction', with its focus on a physical 'dysfunction' of the penis, has virtually replaced the use of the old and unfortunate word 'impotence'. This shift is not only limited to advertising or company-sponsored promotional websites; it has happened in the medical and scientific literature as well. One of the women who looked at Pfizer's Swedish website has also traced the way male impotence was discussed in Sweden's key medical journal before and after 'the age of Viagra'. A thirty-something researcher in science and technology studies at the University of Gothenburg in Sweden, Ericka Johnson has the blonde healthy outdoors look stereotypically associated with Swedes, but she is in fact an American who's lived in Scandinavia for many years. One key finding of her research was that, with the launch of Viagra, impotence and erection problems began to be seen primarily as linked to physical rather than psychological causes, 'a direct reversal of the earlier ideas'.

Ericka Johnson examined all of the articles discussing impotence and erectile dysfunction in the Swedish medical journal *Läkartidningen* during a sixteen-year period from 1990 to 2006, eight years before and after Viagra's introduction in 1998.[24] One obvious change was that the estimates of the numbers of men affected rose dramatically. Another was that in earlier articles the idea of 'old-age impotence' was discussed separately and not as a medical concern.

One article on the causes of impotence published in 1990 is emblematic of the thinking pre-Viagra. The authors stress the need to evaluate biological factors and the man's feelings, as well as his relationships with his partner, his family and his work, and they counsel against distinguishing between biological and psychological causes. The description of the 'patient' focuses on his relationship with others, raising questions of shyness or difficulties with intimacy. Different types of patients are discussed in terms of differences in relationships, and the article talks, for example, about men with anxiety about their performance, or men who have difficulties recognising their own emotional signals.

In the medical journal articles published post-Viagra there are different types of patients described, but the differences tend to be linked to specific diseases—for instance, diabetes, multiple sclerosis and heart disease. The focus is overwhelmingly on physical factors. Ericka Johnson notes that the link between erectile dysfunction and specific diseases may have been stressed in Sweden because of a raging battle in the courts over whether the public purse would be used to pay for Viagra prescriptions. The suggestion is that the way erection problems were being presented in the medical literature was partly designed to reinforce the link between Viagra and serious chronic diseases, in order to boost the arguments for public subsidies—something we may well see happen again with drugs for FSD. As many will remember, such debates about how to pay for the new drug raged not only in Sweden but all over the world, as governments and insurance companies were forced to face up to the new world of 'lifestyle' drugs epitomised by Viagra, and the blurring of the traditional distinctions between common complaints and medical conditions.[25]

Ericka Johnson notes two disturbing trends in the post-Viagra medical journal articles. Not only was the 'patient' presented in a narrower, more medical and less nuanced way, but the discussion of sex had also narrowed. The new underlying assumption, she observed, was that a man would always want sex, but that his penis sometimes failed to cooperate. Similarly, the term 'erectile dysfunction', with its narrow mechanical descriptions of problems of blood flow, had in some ways replaced broader discussions of the complexity of a man's sexuality within the context of his wider relationships.

For men experiencing sexual difficulties, there is no doubt a very positive side to moving away from using the term 'impotence'. Impotence is a word that describes a person, and can be construed as personal failure, literally a loss of power. ED is more something that happens to a man's penis, not to him as a person. Ironically, one of those who proposed the change to 'erectile dysfunction' at the 1992 conference was the psychologist Leonore Tiefer, who describes impotence as a 'catastrophic word'. However, she says the problem with the new term is that it 'makes the penis the patient', rather than the man being the focus in the context of his life and relationships.

This theme—that it is the penis's ability to become erect that is being treated—becomes much more prominent in articles published after 1998, when Viagra was launched on to the market globally. A Swedish article published two years later stresses the availability of new treatments 'largely unrelated to the cause of the erectile dysfunction problems and which demand a minimum of evaluation before the treatment can be initiated'.[26] The message is that this is a mechanical problem with a simple, quick solution, a fundamental shift within the medical literature from earlier advice to discuss the man's experiences and sexuality with him and his partner. That particular article was written by a prominent Swedish urologist with a co-author who was a Pfizer employee. This shift in how impotence and erection problems were being described and discussed in the Swedish medical journals may also reflect who was writing the articles. Before the launch of Viagra, different types of professionals, including sex therapists and psychologists, as well as doctors, wrote about impotence. After Viagra's launch there was less diversity, with one type of expert dominating the authorship of these articles: urologists.

In her writings about the 'Viagra phenomenon', Leonore Tiefer has also pointed to the importance of the growth of urology as a specialty within medicine. This trend had already begun in the 1980s when she was working in hospital urology departments, long before the marketing of Viagra.[27] As a group, urologists have traditionally focused on the urinary tracts of men and women, as well as on men's reproductive organs. Tiefer has argued that urologists' increased focus on male sexuality in the last part of the twentieth century came about partly because they had more time on their hands as a result of improvements in the treatment of kidney stones and benign prostate problems. Surgical procedures for those problems had previously been a big part of their work, but with new treatments and changes in technology there was simply less surgery to do. Around the same time, new treatments for erection problems started to emerge and, like other doctors across medicine, many urologists soon embraced the prescribing of Viagra and the other new sex drugs for men.

So how well do these drugs actually work? By current measures of effectiveness, Viagra and its brother drugs are clearly a success. There is good evidence from clinical trials that the men taking the drugs are able to achieve erections and have intercourse far more often than men taking a placebo or dummy pill.[28] The difference between the drugs and the placebos is also relatively large in comparison with many other commonly used pills, such as anti-depressants or drugs for Alzheimer's disease. One note of caution is that many of the clinical trials have been funded by the manufacturers. We know that sponsored studies tend to find more favourable results, so it is possible that the benefits of the drug have been somewhat overstated. However, even allowing for that bias, if it exists, the evidence that the drugs work well is convincing.

One of the best tools for finding out how well a treatment works is called a 'systematic review', which involves a thorough search for all of the studies that have been done. One review summarised the studies of the effects of Viagra, Levitra and Cialis on men with diabetes.[29] In total, nearly 60 per cent of the men taking the drugs reported they had better erections than before, compared with 15 per cent of those taking a placebo. Did this mean that the men had better sex lives? Only two of the studies reported on quality of life and they found that yes, the men's sex lives did improve. These were both studies of Viagra. However, taking the drug made no difference to a man's quality of life in general, to his leisure, work or financial situation, or to relations with his partner, his family and friends.

Studies of men with impotence following treatment for prostate cancer show fairly similar results, although only one study asked whether they had successfully had sexual intercourse. This is important, as a man's erections may improve partially but he may still have difficulties with sex. In that single prostate cancer study, just over four out of every ten men taking the drugs answered 'yes', compared with two out of every ten men taking a placebo.[30] Alongside the benefits of these drugs for erectile dysfunction, there are of course also downsides. Viagra, for example, is not without side-effects, most commonly headache, flushing and upset stomach.[31] Some health authorities have included warnings on the labels of all three drugs about rare effects on vision and hearing.[32]

So how do these medicines compare with psychotherapy? Another systematic review looked for any studies comparing drug and non-drug treatments.[33] The reviewers discovered only a handful of studies, and surprisingly found some preliminary evidence suggesting group therapy 'may improve erectile function'. Group therapy involves several men meeting with a psychotherapist, providing support to one another and learning from each other's experiences. One small study found group therapy actually trumped Viagra. While these tentative findings are based on limited evidence, they certainly raise questions about the obsessive focus on blood flow and other physical factors being the source of this problem and pills being continually portrayed as the simple solution.

It is important to remember that these drugs don't work for everyone who uses them. In one study of men over the age of 60 who had experienced impotence for at least six months, Viagra was effective for just under half of those who participated. Success was judged by a single question asking whether treatment had improved the ability to engage in sexual activity.[34] Men with more severe difficulties in achieving or maintaining an erection, with poorly functioning testicles or controlled diabetes and who were current smokers were more likely to find the pill didn't work for them. It is also the case that many men don't continue to take these medicines for very long. Several studies have looked at how often men keep using Viagra and the evidence suggests a large proportion don't continue using the drug long term, and many don't even get their initial prescriptions refilled.[35]

But while some men find the drugs don't work, others are clearly happy with the effects on their sex lives and so too are their partners. In its 2004 survey on sex among middle-aged and older people, the powerful American Association of Retired Persons found that around 2 out of every 10 men had used some form of medical treatment for sex—including pills—at some time in the past, more than double the number in a similar survey carried out five years before.[36] Half of those men were no longer using the treatment they'd tried mainly because it hadn't worked, or because of undesirable side-effects. Of those who had tried treatment, around one-quarter said it had a very positive effect on their relationship. Similarly, the survey also featured women reporting a positive effect on their relationship. One Chicago public relations consultant, married to a man with a chronic condition affecting his sexual functioning, is quoted in the survey report as saying: 'The medication my husband is taking now means that age and illness don't have to mean the end of sex. This is not about pill popping, it's about our expectation that sex should always be a joyous and important part of life.'[37]

But not all women have positive experiences when their male partners use Viagra, as researcher Annie Potts and her colleagues at the University of Canterbury in New Zealand found when they carried out a study looking at just this question.[38] The team interviewed almost 30 women who ranged in age from their thirties to their sixties, and who had a variety of backgrounds and life experiences. The researchers were especially interested in how their male partner's use of the pills had affected their sexual relationships and what the women thought about these changes.

Several themes emerged in the New Zealand interviews. The first was that women often felt neglected in medical investigations of their partner's sexual problems. 'We weren't interviewed together,' says one 60-year-old woman, 'because they seem to have this idea that this is a man's problem, but it's not a man's problem, it's a couple's problem and how the woman feels about it should come into it too.' Changes in sexual practices were sometimes seen as positive, but not always. For example, some women feared that their partner would become unfaithful after he began to use Viagra. Similarly, the drug's effect on some men, allowing them to have several erections over a 12- to 24-hour period, was not always appreciated by their partners. 'He'd kill me for saying this,' said one woman, but 'if he takes a tablet at night before we go to bed . . . we might have intercourse that night, then sometimes in the morning . . . and then if it doesn't necessarily appeal to me I think oh no . . . he's going to try again.' Another woman expressed concern about the drug creating new pressures of its own. 'Here we were with this little blue pill that was . . . creating a tension in a way that I was being seen as selfish if I wasn't just absolutely over the moon the minute it appeared in the house.'

Some of the stories also highlighted the way in which Viagra can become a crutch—at times an unwelcome one. A 33-year-old woman whose lover was 50 said she had originally suggested he try Viagra to be able to maintain erections even when he'd been drinking heavily. 'At first I thought it was great, but now I'm worried that . . . he might be getting reliant on it . . . now I think we're only having it when he's actually taken the pills, and in some ways, you know, I don't even like thinking about that, cause it's like "God, does someone have to take a pill to have sex with me?"' These are just a few individual experiences, and of course women as well as men differ in their sexual preferences and attitudes. However, they highlight that 'Viagra is not simply and only men's business', as the New Zealand research team points out. The drug 'affects more than a man's erection. It affects the nature of the sexual relationship he and his partner share.'

In her book *The Rise of Viagra*, American sociologist Meika Loe argues that as a consequence of the promotion of ED there has been a blurring of 'discontent' and 'disease'.[39] As the boundaries defining erection problems have been widened, more and more relatively healthy men have been targeted as potential patients. Others, like Canadian commentator and marketing critic Dr Joel Lexchin, have made similar observations about the marketing of ED.[40] As industry ads promoted the drug for men with more minor difficulties, the line separating recreational use to enhance normal sexual functioning and use to treat medical problems has become increasingly hard to find.

This shift was evident very early on in the life of Viagra, as the ages of the men taking the drug started to change. Researchers have actually analysed the patterns of use among men in the United States, working with data from large health insurance plans.[41] They found that in 1998—the year of Viagra's launch—the group in the population with the highest rate of use was men over the age of 65. Four years later, a younger group of men—aged between 56 and 65—represented the most frequent users of Viagra. However, it was among even younger men—aged between 18 and 45—that the rate of use increased most rapidly. Needless to say, most of those young men are unlikely to have age-related impotence. This younger demographic is also the age group most likely to use Viagra as more of a recreational drug, both for enhancement of sexual performance and to counter the effects of other drugs such as alcohol, ecstasy or amphetamines.

One problem here is that, by and large, these drugs weren't tested for use to enhance normal sexual performance, and their benefits for this sort of use may not outweigh their risks. All three pills—Viagra, Levitra and Cialis—can be dangerous when used with illicit drugs that contain nitrate, including one type of recreational drug called 'poppers' used in the club scene. Men who use these prescription pills recreationally may also be unaware that even at normal doses, and when used according to instructions, Viagra can have rare but serious harmful effects. These have included visual abnormalities and occasional loss of hearing, which are usually but not always temporary. Some men have suffered heart attacks and strokes, though whether the drug caused these rare events, or they were due to the strain of having sex for the first time in years in men at high risk, remains contested.[42]

Legally, pharmaceutical companies are prohibited from advertising these drugs for recreational use, even in the United States where newspaper drug ads and television commercials are allowed. Occasionally, regulatory authorities will even write a polite letter asking a company to withdraw a certain advertisement, as happened with the 'Wild Thing' commercial described earlier.[43] The US Food and Drug Administration asked Pfizer to stop running the ad because it contained no risk information, included exaggerated information about effectiveness and contained suggestions that Viagra was 'useful in a broader range of patients' than the drug had been approved to treat. For its part, Pfizer has publicly rejected claims it has tried to make its blue pill into a 'lifestyle drug' rather than a medical treatment, or that it has targeted younger men. A company spokesperson quoted in the *New York Times* said: 'Have we gone out and given our advertising agency instructions to speak to this young population? No, we haven't.'[44]

One area where recreational use of Viagra has become something of a health issue is among segments of the gay community.[45] Out of the nearly 900 gay and bisexual men who participated in a survey in the San Francisco area, just under a third reported using Viagra. Those who used the drug were more likely to report having had four or more partners in the last year, to use sex clubs and bathhouses, and to have had unprotected sex, including with partners who were HIV positive or whose status they didn't know. The researchers who wrote up the results noted that the drug was popular in part because it allowed men to have several sexual partners in a short time, and not to experience the erections problems that can be associated with the use of other recreational drugs. Although there was no difference in alcohol use among men who did and did not take the sex drug, Viagra users were more likely to use nitrate poppers, cocaine, methamphetamine, ecstasy and other illegal recreational drugs. In some cases, this combined use can be risky, particularly when nitrate poppers and stimulants are used together with Viagra.

Some AIDS groups are also concerned about the link between recreational use of these prescription sex pills and unsafe behaviours such as unprotected sex between men with multiple partners at high risk of contracting the deadly virus. In early 2007, the US AIDS HealthCare Foundation even filed a lawsuit against Pfizer for what the group believed were ads promoting recreational use of Viagra.[46] However, the lawsuit was dismissed and the case never made it to court.

The high-impact medical journal *The Lancet* ran an editorial when the lawsuit was launched, urging doctors not to prescribe sildenafil—the generic name for Viagra—or its brother drugs for recreational use: 'Doctors cannot stop advertisement-driven demand for sildenafil but they can resist prescribing pressure by ensuring that proper diagnosis of erectile dysfunction always takes place.'[47]

It is hard to know exactly how many of these drugs are taken for medical reasons, how many prescriptions go unfilled and how much is consumed on the world's party circuits, though these are interesting questions to ponder. It is also fascinating to wonder how many prescriptions are driven not by medically induced erection problems or a carefree wish for more sex, but by a man's anxiety about his sexual performance. Similarly, it is worth asking whether this anxiety might in some way be fuelled by the hundreds of millions of dollars that have been spent round the world raising awareness about erection problems and promoting these drugs as a quick fix. This theme of performance anxiety as a side-effect of the drug's promotion comes up repeatedly in a book called *The Viagra Ad Venture*, written by Jay Baglia, a Professor of Communication Studies at San Jose State University in California.[48] Echoing the research on 'Swedish Viagra Man', Baglia also looks at the interplay between traditional stereotypes of masculinity and the drug industry's promotional messages. 'Masculinity is presented in a very traditional manner—through athleticism and sexual prowess,' he writes. But perhaps most importantly, he observes that 'intimacy is seen as something that can only be achieved via penetrative sex', requiring, at least from the male partner, a 'singularity of focus, of function, of performance, of workmanship'.

Twelve years after the launch of Viagra, the world of sex appears to be changing. The term 'erectile dysfunction' has become firmly entrenched, both in materials aimed at the general public and in the medical press. The positive side is a move away from the stigma associated with the word 'impotence', while the downside is a more narrow mechanical focus on the penis apart from the man attached to it. Inflated statistics concerning how many men have erectile difficulties continue to be cited in promotional materials, helping to create the idea that even mild problems require treatment.

This process is most obvious in the United States, where television commercials continue to be a favoured promotional tool. Yet in other countries disguised marketing has been more the norm, via websites and other promotional campaigns and materials. Much of this marketing has deliberately blurred the boundaries between erection problems and the normal ups and downs of male sexuality, so that finding the distinction between them gets harder and harder. But in what way might all this corporate promotion of masculinity and the requirement for an erect penis at all times be changing what it actually means to be a man?

The anonymous Canadian quoted at the beginning of this chapter is very open about the fact that he feels better as a man when he and his partners have satisfying sex *without* using prescription drugs. Yet he also describes what seems like a niggling sense that maybe he should be prepared, just in case his penis lets him down. 'To me it is more like your duty,' he says. 'You want to make sure that if you enter a sexual situation that you can keep your part up and this will kind of make sure that you can. So it's almost like a responsibility as a man.'

Six

Premature prescriptions

We're very excited that the future is with us.

—Dr Irwin Goldstein

It was only 7.30 a.m. but the ballroom was already buzzing when Leonore Tiefer's small group of academic activists arrived, taking their seats alongside the corporate suits and tweed jackets. The unlikely setting for the coming showdown was a big room in a Hilton hotel, on the outskirts of Washington DC. Outside the hotel, the first orange blush of dawn had made way for a mild and cloudy December morning. Christmas lights were already up in the streets near the Hilton, and reindeers pranced among the used car yards and the colourful signs adorning the local shops: 'Town Beauty Supplies', 'Hollywood Tans' and 'Discount Meds from Canada'. Despite the modest suburban setting, history would be made today in this Hilton ballroom. In open public hearings, advisers to the world's most powerful drug regulator were to decide, for the first time ever, whether or not to approve a medicine for the tens of millions of women said to suffer from female sexual dysfunction.[1]

Hundreds of doctors, drug company officials, reporters and consumer advocates had come from across America to attend the historic meeting organised by the US Food and Drug Administration (FDA). In line with the normal rules, a committee of experts had been assembled to assess the evidence about the new drug for women, listen to input from the FDA, the manufacturer and the public and then make a recommendation to approve or not to approve. The decisions of these FDA committees can determine whether a new medicine will become a blockbuster in the giant US market, or will be consigned to the garbage can of medical history. The decisions can also influence regulators across the planet, opening the door to billions in global sales. On that cloudy December morning, the whole world was watching.

By close of business that afternoon, the seventeen independent experts on the committee would vote either 'yes' or 'no' to approve the use of a testosterone patch for women. The small patch was to be worn on a woman's abdomen, just below her waist, from where it delivered testosterone into her body. The corporate colossus Procter & Gamble was seeking approval to market the patch to a very specific group of women: those who had previously had a hysterectomy and were diagnosed with the condition called 'hypoactive sexual desire disorder' or HSDD, one of the sub-disorders of female sexual dysfunction. Better known for selling women products for their kitchens and bathrooms, the company was hoping now to sell them testosterone for their bedrooms, and to make a handsome profit while doing so. In the lead-up to the FDA hearing, there were reports the corporation had already put aside US$100 million for the testosterone patch's advertising budget alone, in the firm expectation its new medicine would be approved.

Leonore Tiefer's team, which included a carload of university students, had booked out five rooms at a small hotel in a nearby town, paying just US$59 a night, compared with the US$159 being charged at the Hilton. Several of the New View group, including Tiefer, had registered with the FDA to give a presentation during the one hour set aside for the public's input into the advisory committee's deliberations. They had decided to get involved because they were incensed that P&G was planning to mass-market testosterone products to women for a sexual disorder that may not even exist.

Tiefer was well aware of the limited impact she'd have at the hearing, but she was at the time on something of a high. She'd just won the 'Distinguished Scientist Award' from an association of her peers a few weeks before. Her acceptance speech at the conference where she had been presented with her award was titled 'Not Tonight, Dear, the Dog Ate my Testosterone Patch'. Hilarious, and sad, the presentation was a very personal story of her three decades as a feminist scholar specialising in sexuality. In it, she explained the despair she felt as a 'humanistic vision of sexuality gave way in the late 1990s to a quantifiable corporate-backed idea of sex-as-function', and how this change had propelled her into an activist role. Feeling that despair acutely, Tiefer was not at all confident at she walked into the historic FDA meeting early on that December morning. Excitement about the benefits of the amazing new sex patch for women was ringing around the world, and approval looked virtually inevitable.

The New Scientist, the self-described number one science and technology news service in the world, had reported just a few weeks earlier that the testosterone patch could 'markedly' improve women's sex lives.[2] Britain's BBC had recently run a story with the headline 'Patch Boosts Women's Sex Drive'. The BBC story claimed that women in the company studies had experienced a '74 per cent increase in satisfying sex'. Wow! Who wouldn't want that? Like much of the media coverage of the testosterone patch and reporting of new drugs generally, both of these influential stories painted a glowing picture of the drug's benefits, and neither mentioned anything about side-effects. But what those reading *New Scientist* and accessing the BBC website didn't realise was that much of this excited media reporting was being driven directly by P&G's global marketing machine. The BBC story, for instance, was heavily based on a company press release that featured the astonishing '74 per cent increase' in satisfying sex. The press release was put out a day or so before the BBC story and distributed by the public relations firm Hill and Knowlton, just one of the communications companies working with P&G to help generate the global buzz about its new product.[3]

Procter & Gamble had been busy for a long time preparing for this day. Not only had it hired global PR companies and an advertising agency to help shape public perceptions and debate, it had sponsored key scientific meetings, engaged leading sex researchers as consultants, released a reporter's guide to testosterone, set up a website and funded the educational package for doctors about HSDD that was already being rolled out at universities across America.[4] And this was all *before* the drug had even been assessed for approval. 'Not an exceptional amount of firepower' is how a company spokesperson described the efforts at the time. Whether exceptional or not, it is clear that much of that marketing was aimed squarely at raising public awareness about the target condition of low desire, in anticipation that at this crucial meeting the company's testosterone patch would be approved to treat it.

By 8.00 a.m., the FDA meeting was being called to order. At the front section of the big ballroom, the committee of seventeen advisers sat at several long tables made into a U-shape, facing a large audience of the public. Immediately behind the committee members, on either side of the room, there were two neat rows of chairs. On one side of the room, the chairs were for officials from P&G and their academic advisers, who would soon be speaking about the results of the company-funded trials. On the other side of the room, behind the committee, were another two rows of chairs, this time for the staff from the FDA who'd been assessing the results of those company trials for several months now. At least two hundred people sat in long rows of chairs in the rest of the ballroom, with big contingents of media, consumer advocates and the corporate public relations crowd. As the committee's chairperson began her welcoming address, a phalanx of television cameras started to roll.

First up after the meeting's introductory segment was the P&G team, which had an hour and a half to lay out the case for approval of the testosterone patch for women. A series of company officials and university-based researchers contracted to the company used slides packed with scientific data to explain the results of their randomised, double-blind, placebo-controlled trials. These trials, required by law, took a large group of women and *randomly* assigned them to two smaller groups so that the two smaller groups were essentially identical in terms of factors like age, ethnicity and general health status. One group of women then wore the testosterone patch attached to their abdomen, and the other group a placebo patch. Both patches were changed regularly for the duration of the six-month trials. Neither the women nor their treating doctors knew who was getting testosterone and who was on the placebo. It was only after the trial was completed that the results were 'unblinded'.

Referring to those results, the team from P&G argued that the testosterone patch was a safe and effective treatment for the 'disease' of low libido. Team members outlined how the women in the studies who used the testosterone patch experienced highly significant increases in 'satisfying sexual events' compared with those on the placebo. A 'satisfying sexual event' is the measure required by regulators, and it is recorded by women in diaries kept at home. Such an event could include intercourse, oral sex and even masturbation, with or without an orgasm. According to the P&G presentation, not only were the increases in satisfying sex statistically significant, they were also 'clinically meaningful'. In terms of the side-effects of testosterone for women, like hair growth, weight gain and voice deepening, these were apparently rare and mild. It was still early in the day, but for those watching the company's confident and sophisticated scientific presentations it was looking increasingly likely that the first sex drug for women would soon be approved.

After the coffee break, it was the turn of the FDA officers to present their analysis of the company's data to the committee of advisers who'd later take the vote on approval. The first speaker was FDA medical officer Dr Daniel Davis, whose initial comments seemed rather ponderous in comparison to the slick delivery from the corporate team. But what Davis lacked in presentation skills he made up for in candour, and he soon had the undivided attention of the entire room. Within moments of his opening words, the FDA medical officer was sharply disagreeing

with the position that P&G had just laid out. He was pointing out that the effects of the testosterone patch seen in the
company's trials were actually small when compared with the
effects of the placebo. The small improvements in satisfying sex
may well have been statistically significant, but the FDA officer
was seriously questioning just how meaningful they were for the
women involved.

Davis stressed to the committee that there had been a strong
placebo effect throughout the six months of the trials. This meant
that women wearing the dummy patch had experienced measur-
able improvements in their sex lives without any drug treatment
at all. The message contradicted the way the evidence had been
portrayed earlier that morning, and in the positive media stories
that had been bouncing around the world. The company's PR
machine had been claiming its drug could increase 'satisfying
sexual events' by up to 74 per cent. But in reality this figure was
little more than a statistical gimmick, technically accurate but a
misleading representation of the trial results.

As the FDA officer pointed out, the facts were that women
wearing the testosterone patch had roughly one more satisfying
sexual event per month compared with the women wearing the
placebo patch. Before they enrolled in the trial, all the women
were having roughly three of these events per month. For those
wearing the placebo patch that figure increased from three
events to four events. For those using the testosterone patch, the
increase was from around three events to an average of around
five events—which is how the relative increase of 74 per cent was
derived. But in an absolute sense, the drug produced roughly one
extra event per month compared with the placebo. 'The clinical
significance of one extra event compared to a placebo is not
clear,' Davis told the hushed meeting. At the conclusion of his

presentation there was muttering among the large audience, but the seventeen advisers who would ultimately make the decision were giving nothing away.

The problem of using misleading statistics is clearly not confined to the testosterone patch. Pharmaceutical companies and their researchers have often portrayed the benefits of the latest drug in 'relative', rather than 'absolute', terms, because it can look a heck of a lot better that way. For example, some of the popular drugs used to prevent bone thinning have been promoted as offering women a 50 per cent cut in the rate of hip fractures. In reality, if they are taken for several years, the drugs might cut an individual woman's risk of hip fracture from 2 per cent to 1 per cent. In relative terms, that's a 50 per cent cut. In absolute terms it's a 1 per cent reduction.

Back at the Hilton another FDA medical officer, Dr Lisa Soule, stepped up to the microphone. She was to present the scientific data about the safety of the new testosterone drug. Despite her nervous delivery, the content of her presentation was just as astounding as that of her colleague. In short, she showed that—contrary to P&G's position—the scientific information presented by the company was not sufficient to make a judgement about whether its drug was safe for women to take. 'We are unable to answer many questions about the safety of testosterone,' the FDA officer said. Particularly worrying were early warning signs suggesting long-term use of the patch could potentially cause a slight increase in a woman's risk of heart disease. 'We're concerned about the impact of testosterone on cardiac risk factors,' Soule said.

At the time, the powerful regulatory agency and its advisory committees were acutely aware of safety problems with new drugs—particularly potential blockbuster drugs that would be heavily promoted and ultimately used by millions of relatively healthy people. In late 2004, when the Hilton meeting on the testosterone patch was happening, the FDA was already embroiled in several major controversies involving harm associated with prescription pills. It stood accused of failing to protect the public from potentially lethal medicines, and being too much under the influence of the drug companies who funded the regulatory agency. As in many nations the drug regulator, the FDA, is funded by the user fees drug companies pay when they seek assessment of their drugs.

Just two years earlier, a major study had revealed that long-term use of popular hormone replacement therapy actually increased women's risk of heart attacks and strokes, rather than decreasing it.[5] Then came controversy around the side-effects of anti-depressants, and allegations that the FDA had failed to inform the public about studies showing they didn't work in children.[6] Just three months before the hearings in the Hilton ballroom, the manufacturer of the popular anti-arthritis drug Vioxx had pulled it from the market after data showing it too increased the risk of heart attacks.[7] In the fallout from all these scandals, questions about the safety of long-term testosterone use by women were being treated very seriously indeed.

The hour immediately before lunch was the time set aside for public input, and anyone who'd previously registered could directly address the committee of advisers for three minutes. Among the first to speak was an attractive middle-aged African-American woman, dressed in a striking red jumper and high heels. She told the hearings that, after having her ovaries removed, she'd felt robbed of her sexual desire and had jumped at the chance of being a volunteer in P&G's clinical trials. Experiencing no side-effects to speak of, she felt the testosterone patch had given her a noticeable increase in libido. Unlike most of the people who spoke during this hour in favour of the drug, she said she'd received no money from the testosterone patch manufacturer or the pharmaceutical industry.

When it was her turn to speak, Leonore Tiefer stressed the P&G patch was not something like a Viagra pill, which women could take when they felt like having sex. Rather, the testosterone would be ingested continually into their bodies, potentially for a very long time. 'This is not a glass of chardonnay,' she told the public hearings, 'but it's going to be marketed like Viagra.' In her view, the company's six-month trials were grossly inadequate to assess the drug's impacts. She argued that any decision about approving the testosterone patch should be postponed until larger, longer studies were done—a theme echoed by others opposing approval.

In his three-minute address to the committee, high-profile health advocate Dr Sid Wolfe also focused on safety issues. Wolfe was from Public Citizen, the Washington DC–based consumer watchdog that Ralph Nader helped to set up, specialising in medical matters and drug safety. He referred to scientific evidence suggesting that testosterone use could increase a woman's risk of both heart disease and breast cancer, and urged the committee not to approve the patch. Dr Wolfe, who had been sitting next to Tiefer throughout the hearings, ended his short presentation by saying that a large proportion of women with decreased desire could respond positively to counselling. He warned that the complexity of their problems might be 'glossed over' with the simple prescription of a medicated patch.

One of the biggest names speaking for the drug during the public input on the day was Professor Ray Rosen. Again, he and his old friend Leonore Tiefer somehow found themselves on opposite sides of the debate. Disclosing that he'd had financial relationships with several drug companies, including P&G, the influential Rosen said the company had done an excellent job in its application for regulatory approval.

As the meeting broke for lunch and the crowds poured out of the Hilton ballroom, there was still no sign of how members of the powerful committee were thinking, or how they would vote. For the media, a story that looked like it would be a historic drug approval was turning into a much more compelling battle over the risks and benefits of sex drugs for women, and the busy reporters covering the event didn't get too many moments even for a sandwich. For P&G staff, their billion-dollar blockbuster was hanging in the balance, and the confidence previously exhibited by some members of the team was visibly waning. For researchers like Ray Rosen, there was also a lot at stake. For a number of years he and his colleagues had been working towards a day like this, organising meetings, writing articles, producing surveys, designing questionnaires and overseeing educational programs. Certainly much of that activity had been sponsored by drug companies, but for Rosen the primary desire was to see women who needed them offered safe and effective treatments for their sexual problems. The question, still unanswered, was whether the testosterone patch was actually safe or effective.

From Leonore Tiefer's perspective, an FDA approval of the patch would be a devastating but not unexpected blow, an official acceptance that FSD was a genuine 'disease' and a green light for future approvals of sex drugs for women. But during her lunch break she was far too busy to be reflecting on these weighty matters. She was caught up with interviews by journalists from the major newspapers, the network television channels and the business wires, all hungry for comment on the day's deliberations so far. One thing was clear: the New View campaign—by now involving a diverse group of doctors and nurses, academics and practitioners, students and professors—was growing in stature. Its rejection of the notion of a widespread dysfunction, and its alternative approach to women's sexual difficulties, were becoming very much part of the mainstream debate. The gregarious New Yorker with the disarming sense of humour was being interviewed by everyone.

Another of the women being interviewed by the hungry media in the packed corridors outside the Hilton ballroom was the 51-year-old whose libido had been increased by testosterone. To make her story even more credible and appealing, apparently she was there entirely independently of P&G. Or was she? Present during the media interviews with the 51-year-old was a smartly dressed younger woman who claimed, when asked, to be simply a friend. On further questioning from a reporter about who she worked for, the smartly dressed young woman literally ran away down the hotel corridor to hide. The incident was both amusing and intriguing, and the reporter became more curious about finding out the identity of the mystery runaway. It was only after cornering a colleague of the young woman, and repeated questioning, that it emerged she was part of the P&G public relations team, helping to facilitate the media interviews. In the grand scheme of things, the incident was a very small attempt to hide the company's role in the public appearances of a happy patient. But in the context of any analysis of pharmaceutical promotion, here was an example—albeit a crude and clumsy one—of the widely employed tactic of trying to work with independent 'third parties' who make public comments that are in tune with corporate marketing messages.

Testosterone was, of course, not the only drug in the race to be the first approved sexual medicine for women. Researchers had been testing Viagra for women since the 1990s, and enthusiastic findings had soon emerged. A pilot study was published out of Boston by the indefatigable Dr Irwin Goldstein and some of his colleagues.[8] Their small study of 48 women measured the drug's effects on physiological changes in blood flow, lubrication and vaginal pressure, as well as the women's subjective feelings about how the blue pill affected their sexuality.

Goldstein and his colleagues found that six weeks' home use of Viagra appeared to significantly improve problems of desire, arousal, orgasm and pain, as well as physical measures like lubrication and blood flow. However, the study also uncovered high levels of side-effects, with 63 per cent of women reporting mild headaches, 54 per cent experiencing facial flushing, and 16 per cent having 'visual changes'. While the researchers were optimistic about the drug, and looked forward to the findings from larger studies, they also acknowledged the differences between men and women when it came to sex. 'The context in which a woman experiences her sexuality is equally important, if not more, than the physiologic outcome,' they wrote in a journal article about their study, adding that 'these emotional/relational issues need to be addressed'.

A year after the pilot study, in 2002, the results of a much bigger Viagra study were published, this time involving almost 800 women from around the world. This time there was a control group of women who were taking a placebo.[9] Three of the five key authors were employees of Pfizer, Viagra's manufacturer, which also funded the study. The lead author was Dr Rosemary Basson, a doctor based out of Vancouver General Hospital in Canada. At the end of three months of treatment, women in the study were asked two key questions: 'Did treatment improve physical response during sexual activity?' and 'Did treatment improve ability to participate in sexual intercourse?'

The results (shown in the box below) were almost identical for the women taking the dummy pill and the women taking Viagra, with similar proportions of woman answering yes to both questions. And it didn't make any difference what age the woman was, whether she was pre- or post-menopausal, whether she was taking hormone replacement or not. As with the testosterone studies analysed by the FDA, here was evidence of a very strong placebo response. On key measures used in the trial, including the Pfizer-funded questionnaire, there were no significant differences between the group of women taking the dummy pill and the group of women taking the real pill. So while Viagra may well have been enhancing blood flow to the women's genitals and other physiological processes, it did not seem to be improving the way they perceived their sex lives any more than a placebo could. The authors concluded that: 'Better understanding of the common disconnection between mind and genital response in large numbers of women with arousal disorders is greatly needed.'

Results from Pfizer-funded Viagra study in women

Did treatment improve physical response during sexual activity?
Post-menopausal women
Placebo: 44 per cent said yes
Viagra: 43 per cent said yes

Pre-menopausal women or those taking hormones
Placebo: 45 per cent said yes
Viagra: 43 per cent said yes

Did treatment improve ability to participate in sexual intercourse?

Post-menopausal women
Placebo: 42 per cent said yes
Viagra: 41 per cent said yes

Pre-menopausal women or those taking hormones
Placebo: 33 per cent said yes
Viagra: 31 per cent said yes

Importantly, this study also found higher rates of side-effects associated with the use of Viagra by women, particularly at high doses, compared with those taking a placebo. Among women using the 100 mg dose, a third got headaches and flushing, and almost one in five experienced 'abnormal vision'. If the drug didn't have any benefits over placebos, and it produced these side-effects, the writing was on the wall. As the initial enthusiasm about Viagra for women turned to disappointment Pfizer was forced to abandon its trials, along with its hopes of new billion-dollar markets for the drug. In early 2004, less than a year before the FDA hearings on the testosterone patch, the company announced its change of heart. The *New York Times* reported company researchers pointing to the 'disconnect' between genital changes and mental changes in many women.[10] While the drug could 'create the outward signs of arousal in many women, that seems to have little effect on a woman's willingness, or desire, to have sex' the newspaper article said. Pfizer was apparently moving the focus of its research from a woman's genitals to her head, to look more at drugs affecting brain chemistry.

So with Viagra out of the picture, the hopes of many researchers were that the testosterone patch would be the first drug to cross the line and win regulatory approval on that historic day in December 2004. Yet when the advisory committee meeting reconvened after lunch, it was still highly uncertain which way the vote would go. A couple of FDA staff may have made some critical comments earlier in the day, but the facts, as laid out in the company's testimony, were that testosterone significantly improved women's sex lives and that it was safe. However, as the committee began the afternoon discussions and deliberations, and its members started firing questions at the P&G team, those 'facts' were very soon in dispute.

The first volley of questions for the P&G team was focused squarely on the safety of the testosterone patch and its potential health threats to women who might use it. For the first time that day, the assembled crowd at the FDA hearing started to get an inkling of how committee members were thinking, and they were thinking a lot about women's safety. For the first time, it seemed that yet another female sex drug juggernaut may be stopped dead in its tracks, and that testosterone may fail just as Viagra had. As the questions from the committee became more insistent and more obviously directed at exposing the flaws in the company's claims, the responses from some within the P&G team became less like science and more like passionate advocacy in support of a besieged product.

In particular, some of the FDA advisory committee members were worried that long-term use of testosterone might cause some women to develop breast cancer or heart disease. One expert member of the committee claimed very clearly that 'the potential to increase cardiac risk is substantial'.[11] Explaining that even a small increase in risk was extremely important for a drug that would be widely used, the expert said: 'I don't want to expose several million American women to the risk of myocardial infarction [heart attack] and stroke, with its devastating consequences, in order to have one more sexual episode a month.' The faces of key P&G officials sank.

The committee members were not only worried about safety; they were also wondering just how effective the patch was. Picking up on points made earlier by the FDA medical officers in their presentation, other advisory committee members were now seriously questioning the meaningfulness of the small improvements offered by the drug, compared with placebos. One extra 'satisfying sexual event' per month was nothing to write home about. But apart from that measure, there were also the results from the questionnaires that P&G had funded and developed to measure women's level of desire, and their distress. Looking at the results from the questionnaires, it seemed the testosterone patch had apparently significantly increased a woman's levels of desire, and significantly decreased her levels of distress, compared with placebos. But again, while the differences were 'statistically significant', there were big questions as to whether a small difference of just a few points on a 100-point scale was in any way important in the real world.[12]

One expert on the committee went so far as to question the company about the scientific theory behind the idea that testosterone could improve women's sex lives. She was given decidedly uncertain answers by the increasingly flustered P&G team. Another expert, pointing to the strong placebo response in the trials, suggested that women's desire problems may resolve themselves over time naturally without the need for any treatment.

By the time the voting was to begin around 4.00 p.m., it seemed as if the giant company's case was falling apart. But just moments before the first vote was taken, one of the researchers in the room, who had been invited to participate at the meeting but who was not able to vote, made a very important intervention in the debate. Her comments in effect reinforced P&G's position that the benefits of the testosterone patch, despite the appearances of being only very small effects, were actually significant for women. Even though it was only one extra event per month, she said, it could be important in the lives of the affected women. Almost immediately after her comments, the final voting began.

The vote actually involved three main questions: whether the drug was effective, whether it was safe and whether it should be approved. The first question asked specifically whether the company's scientific data proved its drug offered women a 'meaningful' benefit compared with a placebo. Fourteen of the seventeen committee members answered 'yes' and three said 'no'. The company had passed the first hurdle. Approval was still a real possibility.

The second question asked whether the company had demonstrated that its drug had 'long-term safety'. The answer of the seventeen members of the committee of advisers was unanimous: 'no'.

It was now 4.15 p.m., and the final, most important question of the day was about to be posed to the committee. Was the scientific data adequate to support approval for the testosterone patch to be marketed in the United States? The answer was 'no', seventeen times. Advisers to the FDA had unanimously rejected P&G's application to market testosterone to boost women's desire.

In the audience, Leonore Tiefer began to cry with a mixture of joy and relief. Stunned and bewildered by its defeat, the P&G team instantly disappeared through a door leading off from the Hilton ballroom. A number of hours later, as Tiefer's team was beginning celebrations in the lobby of its nearby hotel, the company released a brief statement saying it would continue to work with the regulator in the hope of eventual approval for its drug.

It would not be long before the fortunes of the testosterone patch were turned around by 180 degrees though. Within two short years, P&G had a major victory across the Atlantic in Europe. Acknowledging questions about whether the patch's small benefits were really meaningful, and concerns about long-term safety, the European drug regulators went ahead and licensed the drug anyway.[13] It was approved specifically for women whose ovaries had been removed, who were taking oestrogen, and who were said to suffer from the disorder of low desire known as 'hypoactive sexual desire disorder'.

In Britain, the approval was welcomed with excited stories in the press. 'The female Viagra hits the NHS', screamed the *Daily Mail*, describing how the new 'aphrodisiac' would help transform the lives of hundreds of thousands of British women who had lost their sex drive.[14] But within months, the drug's luck shifted dramatically once again. An independent medical group in Britain published a recommendation that doctors *should not* prescribe the testosterone patch, which was being sold with the brand name Intrinsa.[15] After reviewing the available evidence, the Midlands Therapeutics Review and Advisory Committee— which is totally unconnected to P&G—came to this devastating conclusion:

> The testosterone patch is not considered suitable for prescribing. Current clinical evidence for efficacy is weak . . . The size of benefit found was small, with questionable clinical relevance, and a large placebo effect. There is concern about potential harmful effects of long-term use on breast tissue and the cardiovascular system.

The following year, another independent scientific group released a further scathing assessment of the testosterone drug, again strongly recommending against its use.[16] But this time, the assessment was even more damning. A review in the respected *Drugs and Therapeutics Bulletin* explained that the scientific evidence about the supposed link between low testosterone and women's sexual problems was 'inconclusive'. Furthermore, it gave an unflattering analysis of the company-run clinical trials, pointing out they involved a highly select group of women. Raising even more doubts, the reviewers said that because the women who enrolled in the trials were having on average three 'sexually satis- fying events' per month, before they even started any treatment, it was questionable whether they really had a sexual disorder at all. Restating the concerns of other independent assessments, this group asked whether such small improvements compared to placebo were really very meaningful, and highlighted that the scales and questionnaires used to measure the effects of the drug were developed by the drug's manufacturer.

What was particularly worrying about the results of this independent review of the patch was what the report had to say about safety. It warned that common side-effects of testosterone included acne, excessive hair growth, breast pain, weight gain, insomnia, voice deepening and migraine. While they were con- sidered mild, in some cases the side-effects were apparently not able to be reversed. The review concluded that the 'long-term safety' of the patch was unknown, and that 'unwanted effects are common and not always reversible'. Reporting on that review, the folks at Britain's *Daily Mail* newspaper seemed to have changed their tune. What was previously being hailed as the new female aphrodisiac was now described as unproven, having little effect and carrying important side-effects.[17]

Across the Channel in France, the testosterone drug was also getting the thumbs down from independent scientists. *La Revue Prescrire*, which rates every new medicine approved in France, gave the patch a resounding no vote. In fact, Intrinsa received the lowest rating possible for any new medicine, a 'not acceptable' rating, accompanied by an image of a cartoon character kicking the product into the rubbish bin.[18] Within two years, P&G had sold its pharmaceuticals business, including Intrinsa, to a firm with a niche interest in drugs for women,[19] and P&G declined requests for an interview for this book.

The portrait of the testosterone patch emerging from all the independent scientific assessment was very different from the rosy picture originally painted by P&G and those on its payroll in their press releases, sponsored educational packages and at company-supported scientific meetings—like the conference in Atlanta. It is a very powerful reminder that marketing and genuinely independent science are two very different pursuits. And it is a wake-up call for more scepticism towards those enthusiastic headlines in the media promoting the latest wonder drug. It wasn't just P&G's testosterone patch Intrinsa and Pfizer's Viagra that were failing to live up to the hype. The blue pill may well have been hardening men's erections and increasing the amount of intercourse as a result, but the new sex drugs just didn't seem to be doing it for the sisters.

Despite a decade of pouring millions into conducting surveys of the condition, designing tools to diagnose it, sponsoring education about it and running trials of drugs to treat it, by 2009 the pharmaceutical industry had so far failed to come up with a sexual medicine that showed meaningful benefits for women. The excited predictions of billion-dollar markets were simply not materialising. The main problem was that, in general, the effect of the placebo was proving difficult for a drug to beat in any important way. The women taking the dummy pills and patches were reporting improvements in their sexual activity, often of roughly equal size to those taking the real drugs.

The challenge of the powerful placebo was in fact an issue attracting increasing academic attention. A paper appeared in a scientific journal specifically analysing the power of the placebo effect across a decade of sex drug studies for women. 'Although resources devoted to development of these treatments have been substantial,' the paper's authors observed, 'to date most investigational treatments have failed to meaningfully outperform placebo in the treatment of women's sexual dysfunctions.' In summary, the paper concluded that 'pharmacological treatments for women's sexual dysfunction have largely failed to perform as anticipated.'[20]

This sobering paper wasn't written by critics of drug companies or of the dysfunction. It was authored by two researchers at the University of Texas at Austin, including clinical psychologist Dr Cindy Meston. Friendly and open, with an expertise in women's sexual health, the young professor has worked as an adviser to several of the drug companies testing medicines for women with sexual problems. She sees herself as part of the small influential group of researchers from around the world, often known as 'thought leaders', who regularly bump into each other at scientific gatherings or meetings of the various drug company advisory boards. This group includes people like Irwin Goldstein, Anita Clayton and Ray Rosen.[21] A strong defender of researchers having financial relationships with the pharmaceutical industry, Meston argues that since the arrival of Viagra, the industry's money has funded much-needed research and sparked a much wider public interest in women's sexual problems. She dismisses fears that closeness with companies can lead to a mixing of science and marketing and says confidently that she sees no downsides at all to the relationship.

In regards to the placebo, Meston explained during an interview that there are lots of reasons why it might work to improve women's sex lives. Chiefly, there are the expectations and hopes that a woman and her partner are bringing to the trial. The motivation to do something to improve their sex lives can bring renewed communication between the couple and may well be paying dividends without the need for any drugs. Similarly, the interactions between the women and all the health professionals in the trials could be playing a big role, reinforcing those initial expectations that things might get better sexually.

Meston's comments are reinforced by the researchers who worked on one of the studies of the ill-fated testosterone patch. In trying to explain the placebo effect they found, the group highlighted the fact that all the women who enrolled in the study—whether they ended up getting the patch or the placebo—had a strong desire to improve their sex lives. This may have led to more communication between those women and their partners, leading to improvements in sexual satisfaction even without any effect from the patch.[22] As others have pointed out, such an explanation undermines the very idea that these women have some sort of testosterone deficiency that needs to be fixed with a drug.[23] It also begs the question as to why sex researchers don't turn much more of their attention to trying to harness all these expectations, and try to help women without the need for medical labels and costly and potentially harmful chemicals.

As it happens, the more Cindy Meston has studied the phenomenon of the powerful placebo, the more she has seen its potential value. Describing it as a difficulty to be overcome in her 2009 paper, the Texas psychologist has since been thinking about ways to incorporate the use of placebo into other treatment approaches, like psychotherapy.[24] The major textbook on women's dysfunction—which, incidentally, Meston co-edited a few years before with Irwin Goldstein and other colleagues— also talked about tentatively exploring the beneficial effects of the placebo in therapeutic settings. But while attitudes were changing, the placebo was still being perceived in some quarters as something of an obstacle to be overcome. Within months of Cindy Meston's paper describing the placebo as one of the 'difficulties' for those running drugs trials, one of her colleagues on the global circuit, Anita Clayton, was outlining a plan to deal with that very difficulty.

With her short-sleeved spotted jacket and stylish skirt, Dr Anita Clayton cut an impressive figure as she delivered her presentation in the spotlight of the grand lecture theatre of the Palais des Congres in Paris.[25] The occasion was yet another big drug company-sponsored conference on sexual dysfunction, this one held in the summer of 2009. A Professor in the Department of Psychiatry and Neurobehavioral Sciences at the University of Virginia, she is part of that small group Cindy Meston described, which has worked closely with the drug industry for years. On top of her other academic work, clinical practice and publicly funded research, Dr Clayton has been the recipient of grants from drug companies, working as a consultant to them and being paid to be one of their speakers. Around the time of the conference in Paris, Anita Clayton had publicly disclosed that she had financial relationships with many of the world's leading drug companies, including Pfizer, Boehringer, Bristol Myers Squibb, Lilly, GSK, Novartis, Sanofi-Aventis and Wyeth, along with lesser known companies Biosante, Fabre-Kramer and Concert Pharmaceuticals.[26]

The topic of Anita Clayton's presentation at the Paris sexual medicine conference concerned a subject of great importance to the shareholders in many of those companies with which she had ties, and to many of her researcher colleagues in the audience as well: how to measure success in clinical trials of drugs for FSD. With so many drug trials simply failing, the question of how to measure success was attracting an awful lot of interest. Dr Clayton's presentation had some good news and some bad news.

The bad news—which most people already knew—was that in general the experimental sex medicines for women weren't doing much better than the placebo in the clinical trials. The good news, though, was that Anita Clayton didn't believe this was necessarily due to a failure of the medicines themselves, but rather the problem might be the requirements from regulatory bodies.[27] In other words, it may have been the case that it wasn't so much the drugs losing, it was the rules of the game that were the problem. The best news of all was that she, and the committee with which she'd worked on the presentation, apparently had a plan to fix the problem.

As they stood at that time, the requirements set by regulators in the key market of the United States went something like this. Drug companies were allowed to use their scales and questionnaires to measure the effects of their drugs, but the primary measure of success in these trials was the number of 'satisfying sexual events' a woman experienced, which didn't necessarily have to include an orgasm.[28] If it wanted to win approval, a drug had to meaningfully increase the number of these events compared with a placebo. This was technically called the 'primary outcome measure'. The results from other scales and question-naires measuring things like a woman's level of desire or distress could be used in the trials, but they were considered to be of lesser importance and were sometimes referred to as the 'second-ary outcome measures'.

In a nutshell, what Anita Clayton and her committee were proposing was a swap. They wanted the questionnaires to become part of the main primary measure of success, and the number of 'satisfying sexual events' the lesser, secondary meas-ure. Why? It would have been desirable at this point in the book to ask Anita Clayton that question directly but, like Ray Rosen and Irwin Goldstein, she was one of a tiny handful of people who declined to be interviewed. The answer, however, may be found in her presentation to the Paris conference. Slides shown during her talk showed that if you focused on the results from questionnaires, the women taking the drugs in the trials gener-ally seemed to do considerably better than the women taking placebo. However, when you used the measure of the number of satisfying sexual events, the placebo and the drug produced roughly similar, modest improvements. In other words, depend-ing what form of measurement you used, different results were obtained.

What this means is that if the drug companies running clini-cal trials were allowed to rely on the results of their scales and questionnaires as part of the primary measure of a sex drug's success, then their drugs would tend to appear as being more effective than a placebo, and drug approvals would become much easier to achieve. By contrast, it has been a lot harder to demonstrate a drug's benefit using the number of satisfying sex-ual events as the primary measure of success, as the regulators have required.

One of the key recommendations of Anita Clayton's committee was that questionnaires should become part of the main way of measuring the success of female sex drugs along with the use of what are called 'structured interviews'. This is a change in the rules that many of her colleagues have been wanting for some time now, and it would certainly be welcome within the pharmaceutical industry. Such a change in the rules, Clayton said from the podium of the Paris conference, should lead to an 'improved ability to demonstrate efficacy when such an effect exists'. The recommendation from her committee for a change in the rules of drug testing is no small thing, because regulatory authorities everywhere are influenced by the views of leading experts like Dr Clayton, her colleagues and their associations.

So, given how influential the committee's recommendations might be, and how the pharmaceutical industry might benefit from their implementation, it seems appropriate to take a quick look at the committee members' connections to drug companies. As previously mentioned, the committee chair, Anita Clayton, had ties around that time to more than ten drug companies, on top of her other work. In addition to her own links, all the other four members of her committee had some kind of financial involvement with the pharmaceuticals industry. And the man listed as a consultant to this committee of researchers was actually an employee of the German drug giant Boehringer.

Pointing out the existence of these ties between committee members and the pharmaceutical industry is not meant to suggest the researchers are doing the bidding of the companies that pay them. As has been noted before, ties like this are the norm in medicine, but they are increasingly being routinely disclosed at meetings and in publications because they can represent an important conflict of interest. The conflict comes about because the interests of the patients of these health professionals are fundamentally different from the interests of their drug company sponsors.[29] Sometimes those interests coincide—for example, when a safe drug can successfully treat a sick person. On other occasions, those interests are in direct conflict—such as when a drug with marginal benefit and potential harm is mass-marketed to people who may not need it.

Serious conflicts of interest may be extremely common in the medical world, but that does not make them desirable. In fact, this topic is being hotly debated in many places, from medical student groups to national parliaments. Drug solutions to life's common problems have shifted to front and centre in our culture, in part because the lives of so many of our leading health professionals are increasingly intertwined with the makers of those same drugs, twisted together like the snake and the staff, that ancient and powerful symbol of medicine.[30] Sometimes those professionals become so intertwined that it is hard to work out which camp they come from.

At the end of Anita Clayton's presentation in Paris, one of the first people in the audience to pick up a microphone and make a comment was Ray Rosen. By now he'd taken up a new position and was working with the New England Research Institute, which conducts research and other scientific activities for public agencies and private corporations, including drug companies.[31] In the lead-up to the Paris conference, staff from the institute—including Ray Rosen—had worked as investigators, together with an employee from Boehringer, on a project that was also funded by the drug company.[32] Certainly he's involved in other activities funded by the public and not-for-profit sector, but can the influential Ray Rosen best be characterised as an independent research investigator or a drug company adviser and consultant?

Welcoming Anita Clayton's recommendations, Ray Rosen thanked her committee for a concise and clear report, before making a comment to them about the need to make sure rules in different countries didn't diverge too much. 'In the interest of investigators and companies,' Rosen said from the floor of the Paris conference, 'I worry that divergence between regulators is not in any of our interests.' The way he'd apparently merged the interests of industry and outside researchers in his comment did not go unnoticed within the giant lecture hall. One of the members up on the stage responded directly by explaining that the committee had tried to treat the research community and the pharmaceutical industry as two separate distinct spheres, seeing them as having separate interests and requiring different sets of recommendations.

It is unclear how the recommendations from Anita Clayton's committee will affect the way drugs are tested for female sexual dysfunction. Already the folks at the FDA appear to be open to giving greater prominence to the results of questionnaires, allowing them as a *co-primary* outcome measure for FSD drug trials in certain limited circumstances.[33] If the recommendations are accepted, though, measurement tools created by drug companies could become the main measure of their drug's success, potentially making approval in the future much more likely than it has been to date. The industry would make the drugs, and it would also help make the tools to 'prove' that those drugs work. In this future, a group of women taking a drug in a clinical trial may show a small improvement of a few points on a company-funded scale, compared with those women taking a placebo. If this change is deemed to be 'statistically significant' and 'clinically meaningful', and the drug is deemed safe, this may be enough for a drug to be approved, aggressively marketed and widely used over the long term. Women then taking the drug in the years that follow may notice some small improvements in their sex lives, which could potentially have been produced by their desire to change things, a change in attitude of their partner or better communication between the couple. But in the drug company-sponsored marketplace of modern medicine, the placebo effect is apparently still seen as an enemy to be overcome, not a friend to be invited in, understood and embraced. The main measure currently accepted—the number of satisfying sexual events women record in their diaries—is by no means perfect. But it can be seen as being more meaningful and objective than a scale designed with input from a drug company to detect the effects of that company's drug and label it a success.

Apart from drugs and placebos, there is some evidence, albeit limited, that non-drug therapies can help some women with sexual problems. For example, there is data showing that certain behavioural techniques, including what's called 'directed masturbation' and the anxiety-reduction method of 'sensate focus', can help women with certain orgasm-related difficulties.[34] For problems of desire and arousal a small number of studies have suggested psychological treatments can help, but there is a great need for more rigorous study in this area. Similarly, while non-drug remedies like pelvic floor physiotherapy have shown promise in helping women with sexual pain issues, the lack of good-quality clinical trials remains a problem.

By the time of the 2009 conference in Paris, Viagra was long gone from this particular race and Pfizer was saying it had no current plans to develop medicines for FSD. The testosterone patch had been savaged repeatedly by independent assessors in

Europe and had still not been approved in the United States. Other companies had stopped and started testing different drugs, some research programs were on hold and others had been abandoned. Apart from the Vivus genital cream, drugs including bremelanotide, bupropion and another testosterone product continued to be talked about as possible treatments. The placebo was still wreaking havoc, though, and none of the drugs was looking particularly promising. But among the wreckage of all these dashed dreams, an old medicine given up for dead was set to make a second coming.

A drug called flibanserin, which targets the brain's chemistry and had failed years ago as a potential anti-depressant, was now being brought back to life by its German manufacturer, Boehringer Ingelheim, as a potential sex drug for women. The trials were only just finishing, and the company's unpublished results were top secret. In the summer of 2009, at the time of the Paris meeting, only a select group of the company's 'thought leaders' had access to those results. One of them was Dr Irwin Goldstein, who happened to also have been on contract to Boehringer. In something of a world first, Goldstein hinted during his presentation to the Paris gathering that the new drug was showing 'remarkable efficacy' for women with the disorder of low desire. Here, perhaps, was the aphrodisiac for which the *Daily Mail* readers were still waiting, the opening of a whole new epoch of female pleasure. 'We're very excited that the future is with us,' proclaimed an ebullient Irwin Goldstein.

Seven

Undoing the disorders

We set trends, build consumer desire and shape debate . . .
—Halpern, public relations company

Psychologist, academic and sex blogger Dr Petra Boynton may get a few more undesirable emails than the rest of us, but she was intrigued by the one with the subject heading 'expert advice needed'. Opening it, she was relieved to see a couple of polite lines and a link, which she clicked through to find a full colour e-invitation, smothered in cute little love hearts. 'With Valentines Day rapidly approaching, we want to talk to you about sex', the invitation read. It explained that an important study of women's sexual desire was underway and Petra Boynton was one of a select group invited to take part.[1]

Looking a little closer at the invitation, the blogger's initial interest rapidly waned when she saw the names of the two suitors who'd sent her this special Valentine. The first was Boehringer Ingelheim, the German company preparing the global market for its new desire drug for women. The second was a smart public relations outfit called Halpern, which boasts of having some very sophisticated skills when it comes to influencing the public. 'We set trends, build consumer desire and shape debate', declares the firm's stylish website.[2] It wasn't the first time—and it wouldn't be the last—that an attempt had been made to recruit Petra Boynton to the drug industry's campaign to help sell the latest disorder of women's sexuality.

Like any big drug company with a new product in the pipeline, Boehringer wanted to maximise the size of its potential market by the time its drug's approval hearing rolled around. In keeping with standard marketing strategy, raising awareness about the target condition is a critically important part of building consumer desire for your forthcoming blockbuster drug. In this case, the target was 'hypoactive sexual desire disorder', or HSDD, the controversial condition of low desire claimed by some to affect tens of millions of women.

While the technical definition of female sexual dysfunction in the *DSM* includes disorders of arousal, desire, orgasm and pain, it is the disorder of desire, or low libido, that has been in the spotlight. With estimates that between 10 and 50 per cent of all women suffer from it, drug company marketers dream that this disorder of diminished desire may be the sexual goose that finally lays the golden egg. As we'll discover, though, in the decade or more since the famous Cape Cod gathering the definitions of all these disorders have become highly contentious within the mainstream of sex research, and HSDD as it's currently described in the textbooks and company press releases may soon no longer exist. The excited marketing staff in the pharmaceutical farmyard may well be counting their chickens, or goslings, before they're even hatched. At the centre of this extraordinary fight over how to define women's sexual difficulties is the powerful notion of female desire, described by the Greek poet Sappho as the 'languid fire' that 'creeps through my veins to all my frame', a description echoed two thousand years later by the writhing Madonna, who was busy 'burning up' for your love.[3]

As part of its market preparations, Boehringer claimed in one of its press releases that nearly one in ten women suffers from this disorder of decreased desire. On the basis of that figure, it stated that there was an enormous 'unmet medical need' for treatments.[4] Yet, like a lot of figures in this debate, this one is of dubious value. The statistic—repeated in other company press releases—comes from a study funded by the very same company and run by a group of researchers all financially tied to the company, including a company employee.[5] It is derived from the answer to a single survey question asking how often the women questioned felt the desire to engage in sexual activity. If a woman answered 'rarely' or 'never', and was found to be distressed by that fact according to the results of an accompanying questionnaire, she was counted as having a distressing problem of sexual desire. This group was then represented in the company press release as having HSDD.

According to the technical *DSM* definition, HSDD is a deficiency or absence of sexual fantasies or desire for sexual activity, which causes a woman marked distress or interpersonal difficulty. As a leading figure in the field has pointed out in a detailed history of this specific disorder, it's a definition derived largely from the opinions of experts, rather than being based on any hard scientific data proving its existence.[6] According to this definition, the judgement about whether a woman's desire is 'normal' or 'deficient' is made by a doctor, taking into account factors including her age and life context. Yet there are no objective measures of the level of a woman's desire, and there are no criteria that distinguish supposedly normal from abnormal levels. Hence, under the terms of the technical definition, whether a woman is given the label of HSDD is purely a matter for the diagnosing doctor's judgement. And this, of course, is one reason why drug companies spend so much time and effort trying to influence doctors' judgements, with sponsored medical education and the whole gamut of other marketing strategies.

With the failure of Viagra and testosterone, one idea attracting more attention was that drugs affecting the brain's chemistry might be able to boost desire for women said to suffer from HSDD. Yet, like the blood flow and testosterone theory, the brain chemistry approach also has its problems. While our minds are a critically important part of our sexual anatomy, the role played by individual brain chemicals, called neurotransmitters, remains poorly understood and there may be more than 30 of these chemicals involved in sexual response.[7] Despite the uncertainty, however, it's this brain chemistry theory that underpins the use of Boehringer' flibanserin.

It's still not exactly clear how the drug works sexually—even to the company making it—but it is believed to affect the chemical neurotransmitter serotonin—though in different ways from other serotonin-based anti-depressants, which have a history of *causing* sexual problems rather than fixing them.[8] The company's medical director in the United Kingdom, Dr Charles de Wet, has reportedly said FSD is affected not only by blood flow, but also by the 'stimulation of certain brain areas' that deal with sexual stimuli.[9] 'The aim of flibanserin', offered Dr de Wet, 'is to return women's sexual desire to a normal state'—whatever that is! Echoing grand claims heard repeatedly for a decade now, the enthusiastic article that quoted Dr de Wet described the German company's drug as a potential 'female Viagra', the little blue pill which has produced annual sales in excess of $1 billion.

Such enthusiastic predictions of the mass markets for sexual medicines for women may ultimately turn out to be little more than fantasy if the critics are right, and these conditions don't actually exist as they've been constructed. 'Here is the perfect opportunity to create a disease condition where really nothing exists,' said Leonore Tiefer, speaking from her Manhattan office. 'Everybody has ups and downs in their interest in sex.'[10] It's not so much the drug companies she's attacking, but the idea that you can set norms for people's sexuality and desire. 'The standard to which we're trying to adhere is arbitrary and too high. Expecting high levels of desire, life-long, sets up standards that make everybody feel inadequate and creates a market for potentially dangerous products,' she said. Her reading of the scientific literature is clear: 'I don't think "hypoactive sexual desire disorder" is an actual condition. It doesn't make sense to talk of this as a condition.'

Whether it makes sense or not, Boehringer Ingelheim has been hoping to generate a lot of talk about the condition and the enormous numbers of women supposedly suffering with it. The company's press releases have claimed one in ten women have the disorder. Its own Dr de Wet was quoted as saying two in ten women describe some degree of decreased sexual desire. A study funded by a competitor company asserted that the disorder may affect up to three in ten women,[11] while others have cited estimates that it could be as many as five in ten women. The more inflated the estimate, the bigger the 'unmet need' for a new medicine. And, as we've seen with Viagra, the larger the numbers of people labelled as ill, the milder the problems need to be to qualify for the label, and the more blurred the lines between ordinary life and medical illness.

As part of its attempt to meet the unmet need, the German drug giant set up no less than seven trials of its drug, involving more than 5000 women across the nations of Europe and North America.[12] The company has called them the 'bouquet studies', which includes the individually named trial: Rose, Dahlia, Daisy, Violet, Orchid, Sunflower and Magnolia. Yet before its sweet-smelling studies were even completed and published, Boehringer was busy cultivating the field of sexual medicine to ensure that influential experts were as full of desire for the new pill as possible. Where better to do that than at a posh hotel, this time the magnificent Hilton on the doorstep of London's world famous Tower Bridge.

An invitation emailed to Dr Petra Boynton a few months before her Valentine's Day card explained that Boehringer was hosting a two-day meeting of a small group of experts at the Hilton. The stated aim of the meeting was to introduce influential doctors and others to the history and culture of the company, and help it understand how its sex drug might be used in practice. The company was offering to pay a healthy fee of £1000 for attending, as well as buying meals and throwing in accommodation for the night, even though Petra Boynton lived only a Tube ride away.[13] Toying with the idea of attending, she started to have second thoughts after seeing the proposed agenda for the Hilton meeting.[14] The title of one of the sessions was a fairly clear indicator of the real reason for the gathering: 'Group Discussion—Creating a Strong Clinical Argument for the Use of Flibanserin'. Here was a company inviting experts to a salubrious location to build an argument for the use of its drug before the studies of that drug were even published, and before anyone even knew how well the drug worked and what level of side-effects it would cause to the women taking it.

This Hilton gathering was organised for the drug company by another communications firm, this time one called Wizzard. It tells clients, including drug companies, that to communicate messages effectively you need to first understand the mindset of the person who is to receive your message.[15] 'We always make a point of talking to the proposed audience as a first step,' says the Wizzard website. 'We work out what they want to hear and how they want to hear it—we then deliver it in a way that they will not forget.' The firm also claims expertise in dealing directly with the public, boasting that its own team of nurses can communicate with patients via telephone, the web and text messaging. Asked about the purpose of the Hilton meeting hosted by the drug company, Wizzard's managing director confirmed it was taking place. He declined to comment on any details, however, saying the nature of his relationship with the drug company was confidential.

Let's just pull back here for a moment and look at the timing of that Hilton meeting in London. It was September 2008. The anti-depressant drug flibanserin had not been approved anywhere in the world. The results of the company's 'bouquet studies' of the drug had not even been published. Even some people inside the company were still unaware what exactly the studies would find. Yet before the data about the effectiveness or safety of the drug were in the public domain, Boehringer was hosting discussions behind closed doors with influential experts, organised by sophisticated public relations firms, about how to create a 'strong clinical argument' for using a still unproven drug. Remarkable as it may seem, the company's behaviour is entirely standard practice—such is the modern world of pharmaceutical marketing.

While she would have loved to have been a fly on the wall at that Hilton meeting, Dr Petra Boynton chose in the end not to attend. She didn't want to be seen to be paid to 'spread the word' about the company's sex drug for women. A part-time lecturer at University College London on top of her blogging work, and a psychologist who has been involved in studies of sexual problems, she believes drug company marketing messages can encourage people to think they're ill when they're not. That doesn't mean some people can't benefit from clinical help and counselling, but in her view a lot of sexual problems can be sorted out by men and women themselves, without the need for a medical label or a medication: 'It's reasonable if you're tired or busy, you're over-stressed or your partner can't communicate, that you won't necessarily be enjoying the sex you want. My concern with this medical approach is that it starts in an odd place, with this idea that a medical professional has to change things for you. It may be that your partner doesn't help around the house—that doesn't mean you have a clinical condition.'

Based in London, Petra Boynton is part of the New View group, the loose global network of sex researchers who argue for a non-medical approach to women's common sexual problems. It was in fact colleagues from this network, including Leonore Tiefer, that Boynton consulted before making her decision not to accept the drug company's generous invitation to the Tower Bridge Hilton. From Tiefer's perspective, the drug company's intimate meeting in London—together with others like it—was simply a chance to milk experts for insights that could then be used to prepare the market and promote the latest drug. But in this case, when Tiefer looked at the proposed program of that

Hilton meeting on HSDD, she was particularly disappointed to see the name of the man who was to chair it. It was John Dean, the British general practitioner who was soon to be president of the International Society for Sexual Medicine.

Asked about that Hilton meeting a few months later, John Dean didn't seem to recall it. Given that he had ties to about eight different drug companies around that time, such an oversight is perhaps not surprising. What was surprising, though, was the difficulty Dr Dean had in describing exactly what 'hypoactive sexual desire disorder' really was, in terms that ordinary people could understand. Asked during an interview to discuss whether this was a medical condition, a disease, a dysfunction or a disorder, using the sort of language people might use in a pub, the usually very talkative Dean was unusually stuck for words: 'Ah ... mmm ... I think it is ... ah ... ah ... it is a ... it is a ... a ... a problem that women experience ... it, it, it, causes them concern ... ah, it often causes their husbands concern,' he adds with a grin. 'She may have no concern at all ... he husband has concern ... I mean this is a complex social issue. I'm trying to put it into lay language. Is it a disease? No, it's not diabetes.'[16]

Asked why he was using the word 'problem' rather than 'condition' or 'dysfunction', John Dean said he preferred the word 'problem' and tried to avoid words like 'disorder' and 'dysfunction'. 'Why? Because it often isn't,' he said emphatically. Clearly the drug companies and doctors trying to raise public awareness about the little-known condition called HSDD are facing an uphill battle. If an expert scheduled to chair a meeting about the disorder has such difficulty explaining it in everyday language, a new set of words might need to be found.

This confusion around the label for this sexual disorder was obviously becoming clear to the German drug company as well. Not long before Dean made those comments, the company had funded a study specifically investigating how people talk about HSDD. After interviewing a group of doctors and patients in Europe and the United States, the study investigators found that recognition of the term HSDD was low, and that 'decrease in sexual desire' may be a preferred way of describing the problem.[17] The lead investigator of that study was Irwin Goldstein, and the other three researchers were all employees of Boehringer Ingelheim. Dr Goldstein was on contract to the company around that time and was a member of its advisory board, as well as being the editor in chief of the *Journal of Sexual Medicine*, where this study on what doctors and patients thought about HSDD was published.

In the journal article describing the study, Dr Goldstein and his drug company colleagues argued that more carefully constructed definitions, based on an understanding of the common language used by doctors and patients, would improve communication about the condition and set common expectations for the treatment of 'hypoactive sexual desire disorder'. They recommended redefining the disorder in simpler, non-psychiatric terms such as 'decreased sexual desire', and explained that this illustrated 'how HSDD can be translated into more patient-friendly language'.

Here is the entanglement between the medical profession and the pharmaceutical industry in its full glory. We see a medical journal editor on contract to a drug company, publishing the results of a study he conducted with three other employees of that company, recommending ways to make the language of that company's target disorder more 'patient friendly'. There is no suggestion of any subterfuge here: all the links in this chain are clearly disclosed in the journal article and, while it might be a stark example, entanglement like this affects many corners of the medical establishment. But whatever you might think about the closeness between the professor and the pill-maker, one can't help but be impressed by the efficiency with which these global marketing strategies are calibrated and executed, and the audacity of the corporate-sponsored attempts to shape the way we think about our sexual concerns. Within a month of that paper calling for a change in the language used to describe HSDD, efforts would be underway to implement its recommendations. And once again, Boehringer's strategy would involve trying to entice Petra Boynton to get with the project.

This time around, the approach came in the form of an email from a medical journal based in Britain, asking whether Dr Boynton would be interested in writing a paper to help educate doctors. The request from a journal to write an educational article wasn't so uncommon. What was unusual was that the medical journal already had a very specific piece in mind for the educator to write. A brief document was attached to the email with a proposed title for the article, details of a suggested structure and a very clear objective.

The article the *British Journal of Sexual Medicine* wanted written would have the explicit aim of getting more doctors talking to their female patients about 'hypoactive sexual desire disorder', but using 'patient-friendly language' like 'decreased sexual desire'. The wording in the brief from the British journal was exactly the same as that being recommended by the paper that appeared a month or so earlier in the United States-based *Journal of Sexual Medicine*, written by Irwin Goldstein and the Boehringer employees.

Dr Goldstein's paper had also argued that the word 'distress' was an unpopular term with doctors and patients. While 'distress' was an integral part of the technical definition of this disorder, he wrote, it gave the impression of a degree of severity that was not reflected in the common feelings of doctors and patients about the condition.[18] Just a month or so later, the brief sent out to Petra Boynton suggested she might write an article that would urge doctors to avoid using terms like 'distress' because they were too negative. The synchronicity in the messages here is hardly surprising. As the short email she received from the *British Journal of Sexual Medicine* directly stated, the British journal itself was partly supported by funds from Boehringer Ingelheim.

For the third time in less than a year, Petra Boynton politely declined to take part in the German company's efforts to prepare the market for its forthcoming drug. She'd turned down free meals and accommodation for the Hilton meeting, she'd rejected a sweet Valentine's Day invitation to an intimate one-on-one consultation, and now she'd refused to put her name to a drug company-funded article urging doctors to use more 'patient-friendly' language about HSDD. She was in fact flabbergasted by the behaviour of the *British Journal of Sexual Medicine*, which had sent her the brief. She'd received it on 1 April and initially assumed it was a joke. It wasn't.

The German drug company was desperate to court the likes of Petra Boynton because she is an influential figure. Apart from being quoted in the media on matters sexual, the psychologist teaches doctors and other health professionals about women's sexual difficulties. She also has her blog, where she ended up revealing the clumsy corporate attempts to seduce her and orchestrate an article from her. Boehringer responded to her blog with a polite letter explaining that when a drug was still in development, it was 'standard practice' for companies to seek advice from experts and pay them for it.[19] Regarding the brief from the British journal, the company said it had been seeking her contribution as a respected educator, that the idea of a proposed article outline was normal and that there was no attempt to dictate the article's content or use it as a 'vehicle for promotion'. Incidentally, Boehringer declined requests for an interview for this book to answer a range of questions about their marketing activities, including the company's sponsorship of the British journal.

Concerns about what's called ghost writing within medical journals were by this time widespread, but this case was a new variation on the practice. Ghost writing has commonly involved a writer paid by a drug company having a secret role in drafting a manuscript, to which outside experts then put their names. In a memorable case, one of the world's biggest pharmaceutical corporations hired a communications company to write articles for influential medical journals in order to boost sales of its hormone replacement therapy drug. After the articles were drafted, the communications company would find high-profile experts to appear as 'authors'.[20] As a result of a court ruling, several of the internal company documents from that particular case are now freely available on a website that has over 2500 documents the industry would rather you didn't see.[21] But in this case involving the invitation to the London psychologist, the idea, the title and the structure for the article had come directly from a journal part-funded by a drug company. Dr Boynton was expected to write it and put her name to it so it would appear that the idea had come spontaneously from her. Once again, here was a new variation on the old 'third-party endorsement' tactic, where corporations try to get independent players to endorse corporate marketing messages.

While Petra Boynton decided not to lend her name to this campaign to shape public perceptions, how many other doctors, therapists, journalists, bloggers and advocates are agreeing to be wined and dined, accepting the seductive invitations and putting their names to pre-fabricated articles, in order to help a pharmaceutical industry that hires PR firms who 'set trends, build consumer desire and shape debate'? Irwin Goldstein's involvement with the industry is transparent, and something of which he is unashamedly proud. But how many others across the health and medical establishment are helping to spread the word about the latest drugs and the disorders that go with them, without the tangled web of corporate ties behind their actions being visible for all to see?

No matter how big the promotional budgets or how efficiently they are being spent, no amount of sophisticated marketing will change the fact that there is widespread uncertainty about whether this new condition of low desire actually exists as it is currently defined. HSDD has actually only been listed in the *DSM* for the past two or so decades, and it wasn't entered on to the international list of diseases until much more recently.[22] The history of this young disorder of female desire, and its possible undoing, helps tell the wider story of how the definitions of medical conditions can be highly flexible, and the labels handed out to people in doctor's surgeries sometimes simply wrong.

The work of the famous sex researchers William Masters and Virginia Johnson is widely regarded as a key source of the modern definitions of sexual dysfunctions. They were the ones you might remember who came up with the linear model of sexual response, including excitement, plateau, orgasm and resolution. Yet when the pair released their influential book on sexual dysfunction in 1970, it listed problems of orgasm and pain but made no mention of any disorders of desire.[23] Similarly, the *DSM* at that time had no listing of any disorder of desire.

By the late 1970s, however, two American doctors are credited with having suggested there may have been an actual condition of diminished desire, and a new disorder of 'inhibited sexual desire' was added to the psychiatrist's manual in 1980. The justification was the apparently growing number of women presenting to sex therapists with problems relating to their lack of sexual interest. Taking a broad perspective, the 1970s was a time when social attitudes about sexuality were changing, as were expectations about the amount of sex women might want. But under the narrow lens of the medical microscope, the seeds of a new disorder of low desire were sprouting.

Responding to suggestions about a new disorder, Masters and Johnson wrote later that this 'new category of sexual problems' did not, strictly speaking, comprise 'sexual dysfunctions'.[24] Yet, despite the uncertainty and debate, by the next edition of *DSM*, published in 1987, within the section on female sexual dysfunction 'inhibited sexual desire' had been replaced with the new term 'hypoactive sexual desire disorder', or HSDD. The label had now appeared in black and white in the pages of the *DSM* but the existence of the disorder was by no means certain, and the scientific theory and assumptions behind it continued to be hotly contested.

Put simply, the theory flowing from the work of Masters and Johnson, and some who followed in their footsteps, was that men and woman are driven into sex because they feel an initial phase of desire. This approach is sometimes known as the 'drive' model.[25] As the decades rolled along, though, criticisms of this model started to mount. In short, some researchers started to argue that the 'drive' model had been derived largely from men's sexuality, and that a woman's interest in sex was often much more about responding to a sexual situation rather than experiencing spontaneous desire.[26] If the critics were right and the model was wrong, then the foundations underpinning the definitions of some of the disorders of FSD could well be fundamentally flawed.

As it turns out, Alfred Kinsey's team had made the observation many years before that women generally seemed to want sex less often than men, and 'rarely experienced sexual desire before being directly stimulated physically'.[27] In 1980, the results of a study of Danish women raised further questions about this idea that spontaneous desire was the driver of women's sexuality, and that low libido was the symptom of a disorder. Researchers had interviewed a sample of 40-year-old women and found that—unlike most men—a third of the women had never experienced *spontaneous* libido, though almost all women had experienced desire arising from stimulation.[28] But it was work in another Northern European setting that inspired a major rethink of this elusive concept of female desire, and a push to reject the idea of a widespread medical disorder of low libido.

Dr Ellen Laan is a tall, tough-talking psychologist from the University of Amsterdam. For more than twenty years she's been trying to understand what it is that motivates women to take to the floor in the great dance of sexuality. Part of her laboratory research has involved showing women erotic videos and seeing what happens, measuring both their physiological reactions like blood flow and lubrication, and their subjective psychological responses. She's found that genital responses to erotic material can happen within seconds, even though the woman may have no subjective interest whatsoever in having sex.[29] Her results have helped build the case that, unlike men, for many women there can be a mismatch between what's happening to their genitals and what's happening in their heads.

Ellen Laan and others have developed theories that challenge the old 'drive' model, which assumed that a woman's inherent desire pushed her into a sexual liaison. Instead, it is the *pull* of a 'sexually meaningful stimulus' that is more important than the *push*. In other words, it's the context of the relationship, and the connection, that tends to pull a woman, rather than the push from some sort of spontaneous desire. That's not to deny that women can and do feel spontaneous desire at certain times in their lives, and at certain moments in the life-cycles of their relationships. Desire has clearly flamed through women's veins from a time long before the Greek poems of Sappho, and will continue to do so long after the pop songs of Madonna have been forgotten. However, this new approach, with its emphasis on the pull of the situation rather than the push of some innate desire, is potentially less attractive to a pharmaceutical industry, which believes its products can help create desire and arouse interest. When pull is more important than push, a pill potentially becomes much less important.

That's not to say drugs have no role to play at all. Ellen Laan believes that for some woman—most likely a small group—they may be extremely beneficial. She is angered, though, by what she sees as absurd claims that 43 per cent of women suffer from a condition called FSD, and concerned that the ordinary ups and downs of life are being portrayed as the symptoms of disorders. She feels the whole field of sexual medicine has been captured too much by the doctors, and women's sexuality has been misunderstood and over-simplified as a result. Unlike Leonore Tiefer, whose thinking has had a big impact on the Dutch researcher,

Ellen Laan does work with drug companies, offering advice and sometimes helping to test their drugs. 'I'm passionately against the medicalisation of women's sexuality,' she explains, 'but on the other hand I'm accepting research funding from the pharmaceutical industry. Otherwise I can't run my lab.' The value of that research funding, as Laan sees it, is that it allows her to genuinely put different ideas and approaches to the test, including her own.

A key moment in Dr Laan's early career came when she presented some brief results of her work as a student, many years before, at a sex conference in Sweden. A very senior researcher singled out the young woman's work as among the best at the meeting. His name was Ray Rosen. A few years later, Dr Rosen would invite her to the historic gathering at Cape Cod, and Laan would accept the invitation and attend. Like almost everyone else in this field, including Tiefer, Laan is a fan of Rosen. She says that his intelligence helps bring a much-needed psychological perspective to the drug companies with which he works. But she also believes he has got so close to the companies that he 'is actually now part of industry', and too much of his work endorses a medical model of female sexual problems that is itself highly problematic.[30]

'That Cape Cod meeting was the beginning of the academic world and the pharmaceutical industry joining together, and it was the start of a whole new medicalisation of women's sexuality,' Laan observed more than a decade after the meeting took place. 'At the time I was honoured that I was given a forum to present my research, but I had no idea of all the other forces at work.' There's an obvious tension between this Dutch psychologist's emphasis on context and relationship, and her work with an industry desperate to maximise markets for drug solutions.

Well aware of that tension, she says she uses pharmaceutical company money to oppose medicalisation. 'This is how I beat them and join them,' she says with a grin—or perhaps it was a grimace. On the subject of whether HSDD exists, this leading researcher has no ambivalence. 'I don't think it exists the way it's currently defined,' she says firmly.

While Ellen Laan was busy in the Amsterdam lab developing her critique of the accepted understandings of the disorders of female desire, on the other side of the world in Canada a professor called Rosemary Basson was slowly mounting her own. Like Laan, Basson had worked with drug companies, and in fact ran one of the large and unsuccessful trials of Viagra. Based in part on observations in her Vancouver sex clinic at the University of British Columbia, Dr Basson noted that there were huge differences in the levels of sexual desire between different women and across the life span of an individual woman.[31] Problems with interest in sex were, for her, much bigger and more complex than a 'disorder' of low desire.

Like her Dutch colleague, the Canadian professor has argued that separating disorders into those of desire and arousal, in the way that the technical definitions have done, does not reflect the reality of women's sexual experience. Similarly, her clinical expertise was suggesting that desire wasn't something women often felt spontaneously, particularly in long-term relationships. She opted instead for an understanding of women's sexuality based on the idea of 'responsive' desire, a desire that arises from a sexual situation and sexual stimulation, rather than being driven spontaneously from within.[32] Obviously some women feel desire spontaneously, especially with a new partner when a new relationship is starting, but for many women healthy sex lives are possible without it. Viewed from Dr Basson's perspective, women are motivated to have sex for many reasons other than being driven by strong feelings of desire. Those reasons are pretty much common sense: a woman's desire for intimacy, her hope to please her partner or the promise of the pleasure of her own climax.

Back in the late 1990s, Rosemary Basson and Ellen Laan had joined Irwin Goldstein, Ray Rosen and a host of other researchers in an effort to rewrite and update the formal definitions of FSD including HSDD.[33] Acknowledging the emerging criticisms of the way female desire had been traditionally portrayed, in this revision the definition of the disorder was broadened to include not only women who lacked *desire for* sexual activity, but also women who lacked *receptivity to* sexual activity.[34] However, as unease grew about the mismatch between the definitions and the reality of women's experiences, still further revisions were proposed. In 2003 Laan and Basson were part of an almost all-female group of global experts that pointed out shortcomings in 'traditional assumptions' about women's sexuality.[35]

This group wrote that fulfilling desire was actually an uncommon reason for sexual activity for many women, and that desire was often experienced only after sexual stimulation had produced arousal. It argued the model of female sexuality inherited from Masters and Johnson was based too much on male sexuality and what happened to the genitals. 'Having been based on a flawed model of function, the definitions of women's sexual dysfunctions have been unsatisfactory,' the group wrote.[36] It recommended many modifications of the definitions.

Around this time, the results of two surveys of sexual problems in Britain were casting serious doubt on whether lacking desire really should be classified as a disorder or dysfunction at all. One study involved interviews with over 10 000 men and women, and found that while sexual problems were common, persistent problems lasting more than six months were much less so. After analysing the data, the authors of that study specifically questioned whether lacking interest in sex should really be called a 'dysfunction'.[37] A second study, run by a group at the University Medical College, including Petra Boynton, interviewed over 1000 women at their local GPs' surgeries.[38] It concluded that, unlike problems including sexual pain, lacking interest in sex was not something women tended to regard as a serious difficulty. The researchers concluded that reduced desire may be a normal adaptation to stress or relationship difficulties, and did not generally require a medical solution. Given that low desire was allegedly the biggest disorder of FSD, if it didn't exist then the whole idea of a widespread dysfunction seemed destined to fall apart.

The groundswell of doubt about whether being distressed by a lack of sexual desire should really be classified as a disorder called HSDD was inexorably growing. Yet all the while the pharmaceutical industry was ploughing ahead with plans to produce pills to meet the massive 'unmet need' to treat this supposed disorder. At the time Procter & Gamble was still hopeful of winning approval for its testosterone drug for HSDD in the giant US market in 2004, there were stories circulating that the company had a war chest of $100 million, much of which would have been spent raising awareness among doctors and the public about a disorder that may not have really existed. A few years later, in 2008, it was Boehringer Ingelheim's turn to start educating doctors and the public about HSDD with its Hilton meetings, Valentine Day seductions and sponsorship of influential medical journals. But as the end of the decade loomed ever closer, it was the desire disorder itself that was looking increasingly sick, a malady made even worse by the publication of a highly significant journal article written by another Canadian, Lori Brotto.

A practising psychologist and sex researcher, Dr Brotto is also an Assistant Professor at the University of British Columbia. She had worked closely there with Dr Rosemary Basson, who was something of a mentor to her. In 2003 the young Brotto had been part of the team proposing changes to the way women's sexual dysfunctions were being defined, but a few years later she'd taken on a much more significant task. She was part of the small international team charged with redrafting the technical definitions of FSD and its disorders for the forthcoming fifth edition of the *DSM*. Following criticisms about being too close to industry, the psychiatrists' association now had a policy of trying to find researchers with reduced levels of conflict of interest. However, under those new rules working group members could still take money from drug companies as long as it didn't exceed $10 000 a year, and they could still hold industry shares as long as they didn't exceed $50 000.[39] To set the bar any higher may have meant not attracting anyone into their working groups at all. Brotto had in the past done a small amount of research funded via pharmaceutical companies, and she may again in the future. However, during this major five-year project to redefine this condition, her connections with industry were negligible.

As part of that process of redefining FSD, the working group released a series of papers in late 2009. The papers forensically examined the scientific evidence, and exposed deep flaws in the definitions. One of the disorders Brotto had responsibility for revising was HSDD, and her measured academic review of the science of women's sexual desire came to a devastating conclusion:[40] that the definition of this 'disorder' was based on a deep misunderstanding of women's sexuality and that it classified the behaviour of many normal, healthy women in a way that indicated they had a disorder of desire when they did not.

Firstly, the *DSM* had defined the criteria for HSDD as a deficiency of fantasies and desire for sexual activity. Yet Brotto's review of the scientific evidence suggested that an absence of sexual fantasy and a lack of spontaneous desire may be a normal state of affairs for perhaps a majority of women, many of whom very much enjoyed their sex lives. Fantasies, as many women will be well aware, are often used as a tool to boost arousal, rather than spontaneously drive it. Drawing on the work of many others, Brotto argued that the existing evidence suggested female desire was often about a response to a situation or stimulus, rather than a force driven from within the individual.

One argument echoed repeatedly by Lori Brotto is that a lack of spontaneous sexual desire 'should not be pathologised'. In other words, healthy women should not be portrayed as if they were sick. Her review of the scientific evidence was published as an article in the *Archives of Sexual Behavior*, and it doesn't pull any punches, explicitly stating that the danger of the current definition of HSDD was that it classified many women as having a disorder when they didn't.

Most astonishingly, Brotto's article calls for the abandonment of 'hypoactive sexual desire disorder' as a label and hints that a complete overhaul of the definitions of all the disorders of FSD may be necessary. To start that overhaul, the Canadian expert and her colleagues on the working group proposed a new set of definitions, with new labels and new criteria. The proposals require problems to be long-lasting before they attract a doctor's diagnosis, and make far greater acknowledgement of the role of relationships in sexual difficulties—something the New View approach had been advocating for almost a decade.

Clearly pleased with the growing acceptance of the importance of relationships, and the move away from some of the problematic labels, Leonore Tiefer expresses a note of caution in all the discussion about women's desire and the differences between male and female sexuality. While many people involved with the treatment and study of sexual problems believe there are clear biological differences in sex drive between men and women, Tiefer says she and others, including Shere Hite, don't feel that the evidence proves such a difference. They point instead to the powerful influences of culture, history and now corporate marketing. The long-time therapist, who has talked with a lot of people with problems over many years, agrees that many woman don't feel spontaneous desire—but argues a lot of men don't either. Their sexual interest is aroused in response to a situation rather than initiated mechanically by some sort of biological sex drive.[41]

Apart from proposing that we abandon the disorder known as HSDD, in a broader sense Brotto's review was also identifying one of the elephants in the room in this current debate about the supposed disorder of women's low desire. She raised concerns that, when there is a discrepancy in desire between men and women, it may wrongly be portrayed as the woman having a problem of low desire. Which begs the wider question about how often a woman's distress about lacking interest in sex is really due to her male partner's distress. John Dean hinted at this in his comment about husbands being the ones who might be concerned, rather than their wives. One has to wonder whether, if a drug is ever approved, how often a woman might feel she should take it as a result of pressure coming from a male partner,

like the comment from the guy quoted in the men's magazine
Esquire who asked: 'What's up with the female Viagra? Where can
I get some for my girlfriend?'[42] He'd do well to remember that
any placebo effect from such a pill, which is most probably the
major source of its benefit anyway, would likely quickly evapo-
rate if it were taken under any sort of genuine duress.

In Paris, at the grand Palais des Congres, it was the final day
of the giant international conference on sexual dysfunction.
Among the well-heeled audience were the many urologists, family physicians, psychologists and drug company marketers who
had come from across the globe to catch up with friends and
acquaintances, as well as with the latest science of sexual medicine. During the long weekend in the lecture hall they'd watched
a lot of presentations, and like all conferences they'd listened
to a fair amount of professional self-congratulation, which on
occasions verged on the evangelical, as leading figures called
for wider public recognition of the important work these sex
experts were doing. But the gathering had also witnessed some
very significant developments in the debate about female sexual
dysfunction.

First thing that morning, Anita Clayton had delivered her
committee's recommendations to change the way drugs for FSD
were tested in clinical trials. Two days earlier, Irwin Goldstein
had given the world his enthusiastic endorsement of Boehringer's experimental drug when he spoke about it having 'remarkable
efficacy'. Now the speaker at the podium was a youthful-looking
woman in a smart suit: Lori Brotto, presenting her committee's
report to conference about the definitions of women's dysfunctions of desire, arousal and orgasm. Her presentation was

a short, sharp summary of much of the material that would appear weeks later in the series of explosive medical journal articles proposing to abandon some of the existing disorders and replace them with new ones containing very different criteria. The Paris audience was in for a shock.

Drawing on the results of many studies of women's sexuality, Brotto forcefully attacked the current definitions of disorders as being 'highly problematic', echoing concerns that had been raised since 2000 by the New View campaign. Both 'hypoactive sexual desire disorder' and 'female sexual arousal disorder' were in the firing line. The definitions, she argued, failed to acknowledge the important role of relationships in many sexual problems, and instead focused too much on the individual. Furthermore, the definitions attempted to 'compartmentalise' different sexual problems, which in reality often overlapped. On top of that, because of the problematic nature of these definitions, many of the estimates in the surveys of how widespread these disorders were tended to also be flawed and were likely to be inflated. The questionnaires being promoted as a way of testing for the conditions were considered to be useful, but were no substitute for the long interviews necessary to understand what was really causing a woman's sexual difficulties.

Essentially, Lori Brotto and her colleagues on the small committee that had prepared her presentation were launching an offensive against a lot of the standard medical thinking about women's sexual difficulties. Unlike many of the other presentations in Paris, this one was not met by a chorus of public congratulation from Irwin Goldstein and Ray Rosen, often so full of effusive praise for their colleagues. Some among the crowd—including Anita Clayton, who was actually on stage helping to facilitate the session—could barely conceal their frustration. Defending a short screening questionnaire she'd helped develop, Professor Clayton pointed out that its ability to diagnose a disorder was highly correlated with the results from longer interviews, which were not always possible or practical. But from the floor of the conference room, there was a different feeling.

One of the first people to the microphone—a clearly thrilled Leonore Tiefer—described Lori Brotto's presentation as 'brilliant'. She told the audience that this presentation in Paris could well represent a turning point in the understanding of women's sexual problems. Perhaps the pendulum was finally swinging away from the dreams of pharmaceutical panaceas to fix the insufficiencies, deficiencies and chemical imbalances, and back towards a more rational understanding of sexual problems in the context of human relationships and the broader culture. Tiefer's impassioned comments, often tolerated with gritted teeth at these sorts of very medically oriented meetings, were welcomed this time with a hearty round of applause from many in the audience. What was becoming very clear on that summer's day in Paris was the enormous chasm between women's actual experience of sexual difficulties and the constructed definitions of the disorders of 'female sexual dysfunction' favoured by the pharmaceutical companies.

For many years, the industry's marketing plans had relied on the assumption that the 'disorder' of low desire was a common and under-recognised condition, and that the unmet need for treatments could be fixed in part by its drugs. Now, from a brightly lit stage within the mainstream of medical thinking, the disorder appeared to be unravelling. Influential experts were questioning the disorder's definition and claiming that the estimates of how many women suffered it had been exaggerated. 'This entity as we have previously defined it may not be any more,' observed Brotto in an interview a few weeks after the conference, just days before her landmark article appeared, recommending that HSDD be abandoned.[43] This widening gap between women's experience and marketing-driven science was much broader than just the disorder of low desire, HSDD. 'Female sexual arousal disorder', or FSAD—the condition Darby Stephens' company had been hoping to target with its genital cream—was also now facing possible extinction, with plans to dissolve it into a newly merged interest and arousal disorder, requiring symptoms to be more severe and last for more than six months. The very notion of a widespread medical dysfunction affecting up to half of all women—promoted widely for almost a decade—was now fundamentally being challenged. And in a very practical way the new developments raised a fascinating question for the health authorities who would soon have to assess the German company's new drug. How on earth could a national drug regulator approve a drug that had been tested for a disorder that may soon no longer exist?

But that wasn't the only problem facing the German drug company. By the end of 2009, the company had made publicly available the first snapshots of findings from the studies of its beloved flibanserin. If you looked at the results from the questionnaires and scales, the drug had apparently significantly improved a woman's levels of desire and reduced her levels of distress compared with the placebo. But if you looked at the number of 'satisfying sexual events', it was a more complicated story. In the trials conducted in Europe, the drug was unable to significantly improve this main measure of success, compared with a placebo. In the United States, the drug offered a benefit over and above the placebo of less than one event per month.

When the trials from both continents were combined, the drug did beat the placebo in terms of statistical significance, but only just. The size of that win was less than one event per month, or 0.7 of a satisfying sexual event, to be precise.[44]

According to the company's material, the most common side-effects in the six-month-long studies were dizziness, nausea, fatigue, somnolence and insomnia causing around one in seven women taking flibanserin to drop out of the trials. Importantly, these figures all came from tiny abstracts of results from studies whose investigators included company employees. The complete results had not yet been published in peer-reviewed medical journals, and the data had not been exposed to the full glare of public scrutiny. When the results were finally assessed by independent authorities, a very different picture would emerge.

In mid-2010, an advisory committee to the United States Food and Drug Administration would meet to debate Boehringer's application to market flibanserin for HSDD. In the weeks leading up to the meeting, the company unleashed an aggressive marketing campaign promoting the twin ideas that one in ten women suffered HSDD, and that this condition was often caused by problems with women's brains. In the United States the company hired high-profile health professionals and a former *Playboy* model television celebrity to help spread the word about this 'unmet need'. In Australia the company courted leading sex experts, flying them to an all-expenses paid love-in in Sydney and offering them A$1000 each for their trouble. But a lot of that money may well have been wasted. On 18 June, the committee of eleven advisers unanimously rejected flibanserin, finding it lacked compelling benefits, yet carried significant side-effects.

A damning analysis of the company's data prepared by staff

inside the Food and Drug Administration revealed the drug had actually failed to improve women's desire levels compared to placebo, as measured by an electronic diary, the pre-arranged method of measurement. This meant that neither of the two key studies in North America 'met the agreed-upon criteria for success in establishing the efficacy of flibanserin for the treatment of HSDD.' [45] More alarming still, the regulator's analysis uncovered an 'increased frequency' of 'significant adverse events' including depression, accidental injury and fainting, on top of the other side-effects. Remember, this was the same drug described as having 'remarkable' benefits, just a year before at the conference in Paris, where Lori Brotto had delivered her devastating critique.

Sitting up on stage at that conference as a member of the international committee that produced Brotto's powerful presentation was her colleague Ellen Laan, who had come down from Amsterdam to Paris for the meeting. Listening to the presentation, Laan was sensing the tide finally turning against the narrow medicalisation of women's sexual problems. From where she was sitting, the 43 per cent figure looked like it would soon be history, and future estimates of the numbers of women with genuine problems would be far lower. The way she saw it, most women's sexual problems are not caused by insufficient blood flow, deficiencies of hormones or chemical imbalances in the brain to be fixed with failed anti-depressants. They are caused by ignorance and inhibition, a lack of adequate stimulation or attention, and myriad other factors due to relationships, religions, societies and cultures. 'Probably the best cure for women's sexual problems is helping women to allow themselves to be sexual,' she observed, 'and to work on the circumstances that may help them to be so.'[46]

Eight

Looking ahead

... in sexuality will always be materialised the tension, the anguish, the joy, the frustration, and the triumph of existence.

—*Simone de Beauvoir, 1953*[1]

If you travel across the vast Australian continent these days, along with the bouncing kangaroos and big skies up ahead along the highway you can't miss the giant billboards selling sex. 'Making Love? Do it Longer' the signs shout in massive red letters. They also provide the telephone number of the Advanced Medical Institute, the company behind the advertisements, which offers consultations with a doctor and the possibility of a quick prescription. Having targeted men with problems like premature ejaculation for more than a decade, the company was now apparently planning to target women with slogans including 'Stop faking, get real'.[2] The institute's chief executive, Dr Jack Vaisman, has been quoted as saying that over 60 per cent of women never experience an orgasm during intercourse. 'My question is, do they need help or do we let them suffer?' he asked. With his sales expanding into Asia and Europe, the medical entrepreneur may well have a big future ahead of him, but his comments on female sexuality appear to be about a century out of date.

We've known for many decades that, despite the seeds of misunderstanding sown by Sigmund Freud, many women—perhaps most—reach climax via the clitoris, and that a lack of adequate stimulation during intercourse might explain a lot of female dissatisfaction, rather than some condition called frigidity or more recently FSD. But the medical marketplace requires a condition that needs to be treated, and the bigger that condition the better.

According to the high-profile Advanced Medical Institute, if your 'desire to have sex is low' and you're distressed about it, you may have FSD, which affects 'four in ten women'—a reference to the 43 per cent figure.[3] Those statements were on the website in 2010 despite the 43 per cent figure having been by then so widely dismissed. The battle over how to define and deal with women's everyday sexual difficulties is by no means over, and the flood of marketing is only just beginning.

Yet, as we've seen, the marketing of the new disease is facing a major obstacle in the form of the New View campaign initiated by Leonore Tiefer and her colleagues back in 2000. In what has become the latest case study in civil society challenging unhealthy corporate marketing, this grass-roots activism with a generous dose of humour has been breeding a pandemic of scepticism towards the new sexual disorders. With list-serves, media appearances and presentations at local meetings in towns and cities all over the world, the New View is exposing the pharmaceutical industry's involvement in sponsoring the construction of this new condition, and proposing an alternative perspective on women's sexual problems. After five years hard at it, at the group's second international conference in Canada in 2005 Dr Tiefer was planning to shut down the campaign and declare victory. Instead, she and her colleagues chose to open new fronts in the battle. Recently, they have taken on the rise of cosmetic genital surgery and promotion of the 'designer vagina', with small street protests in Manhattan reported in the pages of *Time* magazine, no less.

At the same time, Leonore Tiefer's old adversary Irwin Goldstein has moved west, parting ways with Boston University and eventually landing in San Diego, where he runs a sexual medicine clinic on the grounds of a private hospital and has a position with the University of California.[4] Drawing from the famous 1999 journal article, his clinic website still stated in 2010 that 'Sexual dysfunction occurs in 43% of women'. With regard to treatment, his clinic advocates a multidisciplinary approach, including sex therapy, diet changes and medicines, including Viagra and the other drugs that can enhance blood flow. Even though these drugs haven't been approved to be marketed to women, doctors can legally prescribe them because they are already available for men. Recognising a lifelong contribution to the field, in 2009 Dr Goldstein won a gold medal awarded by the World Association for Sexual Health. His acceptance speech, available on the web, is titled 'From Vision to Reality'.[5]

Ray Rosen, a colleague to both Goldstein and Tiefer, has also moved west, though he works with the New England Research Institute. Like the others, he has been keeping busy promoting his own vision of how to improve women's sex lives. As part of that vision the psychologist has in fact suggested a whole new way of thinking about women's sexuality, a new 'paradigm' that shifts the focus from illness to wellness. In an article co-authored with a colleague, he explains that the new emphasis in the field of health psychology is not on 'alleviating disorders or dysfunctions', but rather on helping individuals improve themselves to 'achieve happiness'.[6]

The authors suggest that enhancing sexual satisfaction might be one way to improve general well-being. But in order to research this question, the authors say new questionnaires would be needed to identify 'normal' levels of sexual satisfaction and function in women. And with new tools in place, that could then open the door to testing the effects of therapies on healthy people. 'With the development of new measurement approaches,' state Rosen and his colleague, 'it might also be possible to assess effects of interventions for increased sexual satisfaction and pleasure in non-dysfunctional women.' It is hard not to sense a parallel here with the successful marketing of Viagra to men, in which the line between treating a dysfunction and recreational use for the non-dysfunctional has become increasingly blurred. If interventions—including drugs—were assessed in non-dysfunctional women, a possibility tentatively raised by this article, presumably the potential markets for medicines could expand exponentially. The work for the article was funded in part by an 'unrestricted grant' from one of the biggest healthcare companies on the planet, which is also a major pharmaceutical manufacturer.

As has been stressed repeatedly through this book, the mere fact of a financial relationship between a health professional and a company does not mean that individual's work is compromised. Indeed such relationships are the norm within the medical establishment—but therein lies the problem. Drug companies now fund so much of what happens within health care that there's a growing fear the focus in research, education and practice is too often on narrow chemical solutions to life's complex challenges. As we've seen, behind your doctor's decision to offer you a medical label and a medication is a global web of entanglement so vast it's invisible to the naked eye. But that web is itself the subject of increasing scientific scrutiny, as researchers try to assess the impact of everything from the presence of seductive sales representatives in the doctor's surgery to the company funding of clinical trials.

While individual links may not necessarily influence a researcher, there is growing evidence that, looked at in its totality, this web of influence may well be distorting medical science in the most profound way. At a research level, trials funded by drug companies are more likely to find favourable results for sponsors' products, leading to a 'systematic bias' in the medical literature that overstates the benefits of drugs and underplays their harms.[7] At the level of education, in some nations drug and device companies fund at least half of the seminars where our doctors undertake their ongoing professional development, with strong anecdotal evidence that sponsors sometimes influence these activities in important but often hidden ways.[8] At the level of practice, studies have shown that doctors who accept gifts, and expose themselves to marketing in its many forms, tend to more often prescribe the latest and most expensive drugs, which may not always be in the interests of their patients or the public purse.[9] So strong is the accumulating evidence that the calls for fundamental reform are no longer coming just from grass-roots activists like the New View, No Free Lunch and Healthy Scepticism.[10] Powerful voices from within the heart of mainstream medicine are now calling for a much greater transparency in the relationship, and much greater independence between health professionals and the industries whose products those professionals prescribe.

One of the most important proposals for a clean-up emerged in Washington, DC in 2009.[11] It came from the influential Institute of Medicine, a group that works under the umbrella of the National Academies of Science, advising the nation on health matters. The report, called *Conflict of Interest in Medical Research, Education, and Practice,* argues that collaborations between doctors and drug makers can benefit society through discovery and development of new treatments. However, it says that the many financial relationships between the two groups present 'the risk of undue influence' on doctors' judgements, and may 'jeopardise' the integrity of scientific investigations, the objectivity of medical education, patient care and public trust.

The Institute of Medicine report calls for a range of reforms to bring a more healthy independence into this relationship, starting with new laws that would force full disclosure of every form of financial tie that industry has with doctors, researchers, medical schools, educational providers, professional associations and patient advocacy groups. It also wants an end to all the gifts and meals, and a fresh approach to medical education that ideally would be free of industry influence. Significantly, the report recommends that clinical guidelines—which can have such a powerful influence over how doctors treat their patients—should not be sponsored by drug companies, and that doctors with financial ties to industry should be excluded from the panels that write guidelines. Presumably the same rules should apply to the panels that define and redefine diseases. The aim is not just to get more public disclosure of these relationships; where those relationships are deemed to be inappropriate, disentanglement is the goal.

Other high-profile reports have gone even further, with one group calling for a comprehensive ban on drug companies funding doctors' education, phased in over five years;[12] indeed, some universities are already making tentative steps in this direction. Similarly, a landmark article in the *Journal of the American Medical Association*, written by an impressive group including its editor in chief, has called for medical associations to dramatically wind back their reliance on money from drug and device makers, for conferences, guidelines and other activities.[13] To prevent the appearance or reality of 'undue industry influence', the group maintains that many doctors' organisations would have to transform the way they work, and if necessary drop some of their activities: 'To maintain integrity, sacrifice may be required.' Nevertheless, they argue, such dramatic cuts in drug company sponsorship would be in the best interests of doctors and the larger society.

Across the Atlantic in London, the editor of the *British Medical Journal*, Dr Fiona Godlee, has also called for a radical change in the status quo, and urged doctors to take the lead. In a short but searing article titled 'Doctors, Patients and the Drug Industry', Dr Godlee discusses the way drugs are promoted under the guise of science and education, and argues that doctors should now say no to all gifts and hospitality, refuse to be guest or ghost authors, fund their own education, decline to take on the role of paid 'key opinion leaders' and ensure that research and clinical collaborations are transparent and unbiased.[14] For the senior specialists who work closely with industry, Dr Godlee has a very pointed message: 'Key opinion leaders, your time is up.'[15] Senior editors calling for change is one thing, but new laws are another matter entirely.

As *Sex, Lies and Pharmaceuticals* goes to print, the US congress has just passed legislation known as the *Physicians Payment Sunshine Act* as part of the giant healthcare reform package.[16] Developed by both sides of politics, the new law is designed to force drug and device makers to reveal every single payment to every single doctor: every lunch, dinner and afternoon tea, every consulting payment, every educational grant, every speaking fee, every flight and hotel room, and every single gift unless it is under $10 in value. The name of the company, the name of the receiving doctor and the size of each payment will be made available online, so that the public can search for details about their doctors. It may well usher in a new era of openness in health care.

The proposed law was introduced originally by two powerful senators, a Democrat and Republican, who say the public has a right to know about all these financial relationships. Democrat Senator Herb Kohl believes there's a groundswell of support for the reform. Republican Senator Chuck Grassley says the goal is to lay it all out and let people make their own judgements: 'If something's wrong, then exposure will help to correct it,' says Grassley, quoting the famous sentiments of a long-dead judge: 'Sunshine is the best disinfectant.' And to show they mean business, the senators have included fines of up to US$1 million for companies that knowingly fail to disclose. Moving ahead of the law, a growing number of companies had already introduced new disclosure policies, which will help to bring into the open the flow of money and influence previously hidden from public view. Pfizer, for example, has recently started to disclose its funding of medical education activities and grants to scientific and patient organisations in some countries.

It is tempting to make an analogy here with that wonderful scene towards the end of the *Wizard of Oz*, when we finally meet the great and powerful Wizard. Encountering that little character behind the giant curtain is perhaps one of the finest narrative reveals of all time. It is only then we learn that the curtain has kept hidden all the props and machinery that have given the Wizard his magic, and amplified the little character's voice into a booming presence. Perhaps when the curtain is drawn back on all the machinery of pharmaceutical marketing that has helped create the scientific apparatus of sexual medicine, some of its magical power might be lost too.

The reforms in the United States are certainly dramatic, but it isn't the only nation moving towards disclosure and disentanglement. Australia has introduced unprecedented public reporting of sponsored 'educational' events—though the names of the doctors attending still remain a secret. The medical profession in India has new rules governing gifts from drug companies and Italy has a new tax on promotion to fund independent research.

At a practical, individual level, reforms like the *Sunshine Act* will mean that, sooner or later, we will be able to search the web to see what sort of links our doctors might have. But until those reforms reach our neck of the woods, we can try to seek out care from doctors who have already stopped taking the free lunches, ceased seeing the pretty drug reps, and ended their attendance at educational seminars where drug companies have input into selecting the speakers. And when our local doctor does offer us a medical label, or a medication, we can ask a lot more questions before making an informed decision about whether to accept them.[17]

But as the rules change so too do the industry's marketing methods, with much greater use of the internet now happening on top of all the traditional methods. As fewer physicians are willing or able to see sales representatives in their surgeries, companies are increasing the amount they spend on what's called 'e-detailing', with estimates the industry is outlaying close to half a billion dollars a year getting messages out via this method. There is also early evidence that marketing is infiltrating the internet's social networks like Twitter and Facebook, enabling corporate messages to be embedded in what appear to be everyday e-conversations. Yet social networking sites open the possibility of new forms of communication, which can also be used to critique marketing messages and share solutions to common sexual problems. Since 2005, the New View emailed list-serve has done just that.

As others have pointed out, in the face of the coming tsunami of marketing, at a personal level there are many things people can do to try to improve the situation in their sex lives without turning to professional help or looking to the latest pill. There are websites and magazines awash with articles and libraries overflowing with books, including suggestions about everything from using mobile phones as vibrators to reading and writing erotica for your loved one. Drawing on evidence suggesting women rarely experience desire spontaneously, particularly in longer-term relationships, author and sex therapist Bettina Arndt has made some headline-generating suggestions aimed at ending the conflict on the sexual battleground in the bedroom. She's argued that if a couple has a painful mismatch in desire, a woman might consider saying yes more often rather than waiting until she feels some inner spark of sexual drive.

This 'just do it' approach has been criticised as anti-feminist, though Arndt maintains it's not about encouraging women to be subservient or suffer through unpleasant painful sex. Rather she says it is acknowledging that some women have sex for reasons other than desire, and that 'if they can get their head in the right place' before they start making love, they may respond and enjoy, get excited and reach orgasm. 'Once the canoe is in the water, they do paddle happily,' writes the sex therapist, based on her analysis of the diaries of almost a hundred couples.[18] In what she describes as an 'equal opportunity' measure, Arndt has suggested that both men and woman might consider the impact of constant rejection on their partner, and make more of an effort to maintain physical intimacy. And that includes older men who may retreat from love-making because of the fear of failing erections. 'They too can "just do it",' she said, 'using loving hands, lips and tongue if the penis is out of action—which many women might well prefer.'

Another perspective comes from the writer Joan Sauers. After conducting a detailed internet-based survey of almost 2000 women in Australia, she concluded that many of them would like a lot more sex if only their partners could do things a little differently, both between the sheets and around the house. 'Familiarising our partners with how to excite us sexually and the proper method for changing the vacuum cleaner bag will eventually lead to greater happiness for both sexes,' she writes, calling for a truce in the battle of the sexes and a move towards a new humanism to unite men and women.[19]

For those looking for ways to improve things in the bedroom, kitchen or other favoured sexual sites, it is worth remembering that in the clinical trials of drugs, simply taking a placebo appeared to help many women—suggesting that a couple's willingness to change may help bring it on. And when outside assistance is needed, there are doctors and clinics and counsellors who can help with a range of strategies for even the most debilitating problems, like pain on intercourse. Being sceptical is not about losing complete trust in medical approaches or pharmaceutical solutions, but rather taking a little more time to try to sort the false hype from the genuine hope. But the milder a problem is, the smaller the benefit that can come from a medical label and a pill, and the bigger the risk of doing more harm than good. We all need drug companies to continue producing safe and effective medicines, but whether we need them to keep telling us when to see our doctors is another question. While many within the small circles of sex research still welcome the industry's role in building the science of sexual dysfunction, others fear an unhealthy merging of marketing and medicine that could well leave too many women believing they have a disorder when they don't.

However good the clinics, the doctors, the drugs, the vibrators or the partner's technique with the vacuum cleaner, as Simone de Beauvoir has written, sex will likely remain fraught with frustration and anguish, along with its all its joys and triumphs.[20] De Beauvoir reminds us too that, while the differences between the sexes can at times seem huge—particularly during those battles over desire—what unites us is far bigger. The fact that we are human beings, she writes, is 'infinitely more important' than all the peculiarities that distinguish us one from the other. 'In both sexes is played out the same drama of the flesh and spirit, of finitude and transcendence; both gnawed away by time and laid in wait for by death . . .'

De Beauvoir's dream of freedom is ultimately a powerfully positive one, foreseeing a time when women are no longer the second sex, having won complete economic and social equality with men. The way the French philosopher imagined it, for the truly independent woman a traditional femininity based on dependence might fade and old forms of sexuality may shift as a result, but new relations of 'flesh and sentiment' will arise and the human miracles of desire, dream, love and adventure will live on. Perhaps we might dream too that in such a world the sexuality of both men and women will be far less affected by marketing messages selling medical solutions to life's everyday challenges, and a genuine science of sexuality may emerge less distorted by the sex drive of corporate gain or the naked ambition of professional self-interest.

Acknowledgements

Ray says: Many thanks to all those within the publishing world who've helped create this work, but particularly Rob Sanders in Canada for his early and ongoing enthusiasm and Rebecca Kaiser for steering this international project through. At the *BMJ*, there have been several key people who've encouraged the reporting on the entanglement between the medical profession and the drug industry, and the corporate-sponsored medicalisation of ordinary life, which has helped drive the book. They include chiefly the former editor Richard Smith, the current editor Fiona Godlee, and one of the best news editors in the world for whom to work, the indefatigable, efficient, rigorous and charming Annabel Ferriman.

Thanks to all those who contributed to the research and worked in other ways on the book, including Freda Haylett—who examined the emerging intersection of marketing and social networking via the web—and my friend and previous co-author Melissa Sweet—who gathered data on the changing nature of our social lives. Librarians all over the world also deserve a big hug, especially those at the University of Newcastle and the library in Byron Bay. Thanks also to co-author Barbara Mintzes, whose expertise on pharmaceutical marketing informed the whole of the manuscript and who drafted the chapter on Viagra.

Thanks are also due to Leslie Cannold, who offered intelligent and timely criticism of an early draft, and to Christine Willmot, who also gave valuable feedback and encouragement. I'm grateful to all the people who were interviewed for the book, or helped with the process of fact-checking, including Ananda Davis, Bettina Arndt, Cindy Meston, Cynthia Graham, Dilek Erdogru, Ed Laumann, Ellen Laan, Erick Janssen, Heather Holst, Jean Fourcroy, Joan Souers, John Bancroft, John Dean, Julia Heiman, Juliet Richters, Kirstin Mitchell, Kerstin Fugl-Meyer, Leonore Tiefer, Lori Brotto, Lorraine Dennerstein, Marita McCabe, Michael King, Miranda Burne, Petra Boynton, Ronda Taylor, Shannon Brownlee and Wendy Vanselow. A very special thanks in particular to Leonore Tiefer for making herself available for several interviews. Apologies to any people accidentally left off, and to the company insiders who can't be named. Thanks too to Pat Fiske and Cathy Scott for the material shot for the *Selling Sickness* film, used in Chapter 3. And a very warm thanks to the wonderful Liz Canner—the film director who interviewed me on a number of occasions for her documentary, *Orgasm Inc.*—for the Darby Stephens interview material and for the conversations when some of the ideas for a possible book on this topic were being formed.

Finally, I am indebted again to my family and friends for bearing with me and buoying me up through the challenging times of the past year or two when this manuscript was being written. Chief among them is Miranda, whose love and support has given me life in the midst of the sadness and grief surrounding the loss of my sister, Toni. And to Toni, whose honesty, warmth and openness have inspired so many of us, I want to again repeat the words we would say to each other on the steps of her Melbourne home, as we would part smiling and laughing at the end of all those sad and shining days: thank you.

Barbara says: Thanks to Jennifer Matthews for her assistance with the interviews for Chapter 5, and to Stephen Adams for his help with document retrieval. I would also like to thank Ericka Johnson for her willingness to be interviewed and assistance with extra questions.

Notes

Introduction

1 I. Goldstein, C. Meston, S. Davis & A. Traish (eds), *Women's Sexual Function and Dysfunction*, Taylor & Francis, Boca Raton, 2006, p. 323.

2 *Diagnostic and Statistical Manual of Mental Disorders*, American Psychiatric Association, Arlington, Va., http://psych.org/MainMenu/Research/DSMIV.aspx.

3 Business World, 'IMS Sees Brighter Outlook For Global Drug Sales', 8 October 2009, www.businessworld.in/bw/2009_10_08_IMS_Sees_Brighter_Outlook_For_Global_Drug_Sales.html.

4 For more on this process, see R. Moynihan & A. Cassels, *Selling Sickness: How drug companies are turning us all into patients*, Allen & Unwin, Sydney, 2005.

5 D. Fitzhenry & L. Sandberg, 'From the analyst's couch: Female sexual dysfunction', *Nature Reviews*, vol. 4, 2005, pp. 99–100.

6 R. Moynihan, 'The marketing of a disease: Female sexual dysfunction', *BMJ*, vol. 330, 2005, pp. 192–4.

7 P&G sold its pharmaceutical business in 2009.

8 Katie 448, http://katie448.livejournal.com/2712.html.

9 For genital cosmetic surgery material see www.fsd-alert.org; for pink products see www.mynewpinkbutton.com.

10 R. Basson, J. Berman & A. Burnett et. al, 'Report of the international consensus development conference on female sexual dysfunction: Definitions and classifications', *Journal of Urology*, vol. 163, 2000, pp. 888–93.

11 R. Eckersley, *Well and Good*, Text Publishing, Melbourne, 2004.
12 S. de Beauvoir, *The Second Sex*, Lowe and Brydone, Jonathan Cape, London, 1953, p. 686.
13 See the Institute of Medicine report, *Conflict of Interest in Medical Research, Education, and Practice*, April 2009, www.iom.edu/Reports/2009/Conflict-of-Interest-in-Medical-Research-Education-and-Practice.aspx.

Chapter 1 Difficulties or dysfunctions?

1   Interview conducted by Liz Canner for her documentary, *Orgasm Inc.* All the quotes are from the same source.
2   V. Parry, 'The art of branding a condition', *MM&M*, May 2003, pp. 43–9; the second quote is taken from Vince Parry's interview with Cathy Scott for *Selling Sickness*, the documentary, Paradigm Pictures, 2004.
3   N. Klein, *No Logo*, Flamingo, London, 2000.
4   I. Goldstein, C. Meston, S. Davis & A. Traish (eds), *Women's Sexual Function and Dysfunction*, Taylor & Francis, Boca Raton, 2006, p. 323.
5   H. Cohen, 'Expanding mental illness', *Background Briefing* program, Australian Broadcasting Corporation, 12 July 2009, www.abc.net.au/rn/backgroundbriefing/stories/2009/2619066.htm. Also see A. Frances, 'A warning sign on the road to *DSM-V*: Beware of its unintended consequences', *Psychiatric Times*, 26 June 2009.
6   L. Cosgrove et. al., 'Financial ties between DSM-IV panel members and the pharmaceutical industry', *Psychotherapy and Psychosomatics*, vol. 75, 2006, pp. 154–60.
7   This suggestion is canvassed in L. Brotto, 'The DSM diagnostic criteria for hypoactive sexual desire disorder in women', *Archives of Sexual Behavior*, 24 September 2009, epub ahead of print.
8   www.fsd-alert.org.
9   L. Tiefer & E. Kaschak, *A New View of Women's Sexual Problems*, The Haworth Press, New York, 2001; also see www.fsd-alert.org/manifesto3.asp.
10 This quote was cited in P. Robinson, *The Modernisation of Sex*, Harper and Row, New York, 1976, p. 27. This book is one of the sources that has informed the material in this section.
11 P. Gay (ed.), *The Freud Reader*, Vintage, London, 1995. The first quote is from *Three Essays on the Theory of Sexuality*, 1924 (p. 287 of *The Freud Reader*); the second quote is from *Some Psychical Consequences of the Anatomical Distinction between the Sexes*, 1925 (p. 675 of *The Freud Reader*).
12 Goldstein et. al., *Women's Sexual Function and Dysfunction*, Ch. 11.1.

13 W. Kroger & C. Freed, 'Psychosomatic aspects of frigidity', *JAMA*, vol. 143, 1950, pp. 526–32.

14 A. Kinsey et. al., *Sexual Behaviour in the Human Female*, W.B. Saunders, New York, 1953. Coming quote is from p. 373.

15 P. Robinson, *The Modernisation of Sex*, Harper and Row, New York, 1976.

16 S. de Beauvoir, *The Second Sex*, Lowe and Brydone, Jonathan Cape, London, 1953, p. 15.

17 Goldstein et. al., *Women's Sexual Function and Dysfunction*, Ch. 1.1. This chapter has been one of the sources for this section of the book.

18 P. Robinson, *The Modernisation of Sex*, Harper and Row, New York, 1976, p. 151.

19 W. Masters & V. Johnson, *Human Sexual Inadequacy*, Little, Brown and Co., Boston, 1970, chapter 13.

20 ibid., p. 218.

21 *Kinsey*, Dir. Bill Condon, Searchlight Pictures, 2004.

22 Ray Moynihan interview with Leonore Tiefer, 2010.

23 Masters & Johnson, *Human Sexual Inadequacy*, p. v.

24 S. Hite, *The Hite Report*, Seven Stories, New York, 1976.

25 Pfizer advertisement, *Journal of Sexual Medicine*, vol. 1, 2004, back cover.

26 P. Abramson, 'Sexual science: Emerging discipline or oxymoron', *Journal of Sex Research*, vol. 27, 1990, pp. 147–65.

27 L. Tiefer, 'Sexology and the pharmaceutical industry: The threat of co-optation', *The Journal of Sex Research*, vol. 37, 2000, pp. 273–83.

28 L. Tiefer, 'In pursuit of the perfect penis: The medicalisation of male sexuality', *American Behavioral Scientist*, vol. 29, 1986, pp. 579–99.

29 L. Tiefer, 'Sexology and the pharmaceutical industry'. Also see L. Tiefer, 'A new view of women's sexual problems: Why new? Why now?', *The Journal of Sex Research*, vol. 38, 2001, pp. 89–96.

30 Email from Ray Rosen to Leonore Tiefer, 10 May 1997.

31 R. Basson, J. Berman & A. Burnett et. al., 'Report of the international consensus development conference on female sexual dysfunction: Definitions and classifications', *Journal of Urology*, vol. 163, 2000, pp. 888–93.

32 R. Moynihan, 'The making of a disease: Female sexual dysfunction', *BMJ*, vol. 326, 2003, pp. 45–7.

33 ibid.

34 Ray Moynihan interview with Darby Stephens, 5 February 2010.

35 R. Moynihan, 'The making of a disease: Female sexual dysfunction'.

36 Pfizer's response to Ray Moynihan's questions, 2010.

37 More on this in Chapter 4.

38 J. Coe, 'The lifestyle drugs outlook to 2008: Unlocking new value in well-being', Datamonitor, *Reuters Business Insights, Healthcare*, PLC, 2003.

39 L. Tiefer, 'The medicalisation of sexuality: Conceptual, normative, and professional issues', *Annual Review of Sex Research*, vol. 7, 1996, pp. 252–82.

40 J. Ha Kim, 'When Samantha took a hit of Viagra on *Sex and the City*', *Chicago Sun-Times*, 11 November 2003.

41 R. Moynihan, 'The making of a disease: Female sexual dysfunction'.

42 S. Hite, 'The truth about women and sex', *The Age*, 28 January 2003, www.theage.com.au/articles/2003/01/27/1043534001783.html.

43 S Brownlee, *Overtreated: Why too much medicine is making us sicker and poorer*, Bloomsbury, USA, 2007; R. Moynihan, *Too Much Medicine?*, ABC Books, Sydney, 1998.

44 E. Laumann, A. Paik & R. Rosen, 'Sexual dysfunction in the United States', *JAMA*, vol. 281, 1999, pp. 537–44.

Chapter 2   43 per cent

1 E. Laumann, A. Paik & R. Rosen, 'Sexual dysfunction in the United States', *JAMA*, vol. 281, 1999, pp. 537–44.

2 The citation figures come from Ray Moynihan's interview with Ed Laumann, 2010. Google search of '43%' and 'female sexual dysfunction' produced 32,000 hits on 9 September 2009.

3 'Bad news in the bedroom: A sex study finds widespread dysfunction', *Newsweek*, 22 February 1999.

4 Press release from Front Line Strategic Consulting Inc., 21 November 2002.

5 E. Laumann, J, Gagnon, R. Michael & S. Michaels, *The Social Organisation of Sexuality*, University of Chicago Press, Chicago, 1994.

6 This section has drawn on many different sources including an interview with Ed Laumann. Also I. Goldstein, C. Meston, S. Davis & A. Traish (eds), *Women's Sexual Function and Dysfunction*, Taylor & Francis, Boca Raton, 2006, Ch. 2.1; K. Mitchell, Sexual Dysfunction: Conceptual and Measurement Issues, unpublished doctoral dissertation, London School of Hygiene and Tropical Medicine, 2008; K. Zucker, 'Sexology and epidemiology', *Archives of Sexual Behavior*, vol. 36, 2007, pp. 1–3; R. Segraves & T. Woodard, 'Female hypoactive sexual desire disorder: History and current status', *Journal of Sexual Medicine*, vol. 3, 2006, pp. 408–18.

7 R. Basson, J. Berman & A. Burnett et. al., 'Report of the International Consensus Development Conference on Female Sexual Dysfunction: Definitions and classifications', *Journal of Urology*, vol. 163, 2000, pp. 888–93.

8 This paragraph is drawing on K. Zucker, 'Sexology and epidemiology', *Archives of Sexual Behavior*, vol. 36, 2007, pp. 1–3.

9   I. Goldstein et. al., *Women's Sexual Function and Dysfunction*, p. 745.

10   R. Moynihan, 'The making of a disease: Female sexual dysfunction', *BMJ*, vol. 326, 2003, pp. 45–7. The following quote from Goldstein also comes from this paper.

11   D. Grady, ' Better loving through chemistry: Sure, we've got a pill for that', *New York Times*, 14 February 1999.

12   Corrections, *JAMA*, vol. 281, 1999, p. 1174.

13   Ray Moynihan interview with Ed Laumann, July 2009.

14   Goldstein et. al., *Women's Sexual Function and Dysfunction*, p. 23.

15   This is drawn on J. Bancroft, J. Loftus & S. Long, 'Distress about sex: A national survey of women in heterosexual relationships', *Archives of Sexual Behavior*, vol. 32, 2003, pp. 193–208.

16   J. Bancroft, J. Loftus & S. Long, 'Distress about sex: A national survey of women in heterosexual relationships', pp. 194–208.

17   R Moynihan, 'The marketing of a disease: Female sexual dysfunction', *BMJ*, vol. 330, 2005, pp. 192–4.

18   Mitchell, Sexual Dysfunction, Ch. 20.

19   Bancroft et. al., 'Distress about sex: A national survey'.

20   B. Marshall, 'Science, medicine and virility surveillance: Sex seniors in the pharmaceutical imagination', *Sociology of Health and Illness*, 2010, vol. 32, pp. 211–24.

21   Goldstein et. al., *Women's Sexual Function and Dysfunction*. Ch. 2.4.

22   M. King, V. Holt & I. Nazareth, 'Women's views of their sexual difficulties: Agreement and disagreement with clinical diagnoses', *Archives of Sexual Behavior*, vol. 36, 2007, pp. 281–8.

23   See C. Mercer, K. Fenton & A. Johnson et. al., 'Sexual function problems and help seeking behaviour in Britain: National probability sample survey', *BMJ*, vol. 327, 2003, pp. 426–7; I. Nazareth, P. Boynton & M. King, 'Problems with sexual function in people attending London general practitioners: A cross sextional study', *BMJ*, vol. 327, 2003, p. 423.

24   Ray Moynihan interviews with Michael King, 2009, 2010.

25   The survey participants were all over 40. These two papers are sources for the following discussion. E. Laumann, A. Nicolosi & D. Glasser et. al., 'Sexual problems among women and men aged 40–80: Prevalence and correlates identified in the Global Study of Sexual Attitudes and Behaviors', *International Journal of Impotence Research*, vol. 17, 2005, pp. 39–57; E. Laumann, A. Paik & D. Glasser et. al., 'A cross-national study of subjective sexual well-being among older women and men: Findings from the global study of sexual attitudes and behaviors', *Archives of Sexual Behavior*, vol. 35, 2006, pp. 145–61.

26 Ray Moynihan interview with Ed Laumann, 2010.

27 E. Laumann et. al., 'Sexual problems among women and men aged 40–80', table Ia, p. 42.

28 ibid.

29 Pfizer's response to Ray Moynihan questions 2010.

30 S. Leiblum, P. Koochacki & C. Rodenburg et. al., 'Hypoactive sexual desire disorder in postmenopausal women: US results from the women's international study of health and sexuality (Wishes)', *Menopause*, vol. 13, 2006, pp. 46–56.

31 Boehringer press release, 'New diagnostic tool helps health care professionals accurately diagnose Hypoactive Sexual Desire Disorder (HSDD) in women', 3 March 2009; J. Shifren, B. Monz, P. Russo, A. Segreti & C. Johannes, 'Sexual problems and distress in United States women: prevalence and correlates', *Obstetrics and Gynecology*, vol. 112, 2008, pp. 970–8.

32 R. Munarriz, N. Kim, A. Traish & I. Goldstein, 'Female Sexual Dysfunction', in A. Seftell, *Male and Female Sexual Dysfunction*, Mosby, Elsevier, Edinburgh, 2004.

33 R. Moynihan & A. Cassels, *Selling Sickness: How the drug companies are turning us all into patients*, Allen & Unwin, Sydney, 2005.

34 R. Moynihan, 'Scientists find new disease: Motivational deficiency disorder', *BMJ*, vol. 332, 2006, p. 745.

35 *Sex in Australia:* Summary findings of the Australian study of health and relationships, www.latrobe.edu.au/ashr/papers/Sex%20In%20Australia%20Summary.pdf.

36 ibid., p. 4 of summary.

37 This section and the previous paragraph draw on Ray Moynihan's interview with Juliet Richters, 2009. The quote is from J. Richters, 'Bodies, pleasure and displeasure', *Culture, Health & Sexuality*, vol. 11, 2009, pp. 225–36. There is a segment in this article called 'Measuring sexual pleasure', which likely inspired the name for chapter three of this book.

38 ibid., p. 232.

39 Mitchell, Sexual Dysfunction.

Chapter 3   Measuring pleasure

1 The doctor was giving a tour of the new Berman centre: www.bermancenter.com. The quotes came from an interview conducted for the documentary, *Selling Sickness*, Paradigm Pictures, 2004.

2 This section has drawn on two chapters from I. Goldstein, C. Meston,

S. Davis & A. Traish (eds), *Women's Sexual Function and Dysfunction*, Taylor & Francis, Boca Raton, 2006, Chs 10.1 and 10.2.

3   Ray Moynihan interviews with Leonore Tiefer, 2009, 2010.

4   Goldstein et. al., *Women's Sexual Function and Dysfunction*, Ch. 10.1.

5   ibid., p. 364. The quote is from Ray Moynihan's interview with Erick Janssen, 2010.

6   ibid., Ch. 10.2. Also drawn from comments by Lori Brotto during her committee # 24 presentation at the ICSM 3 conference in Paris, 10–13 July 2009.

7   Transcript of interviews at the opening of the Berman centre, p. 12.

8   See Goldstein et. al., pp. 383 and 434; also drawing on comments from Lori Brotto during her committee # 24 presentation at the ICSM 3 conference in Paris, 10–13 July 2009.

9   Personal communication between Ray Moynihan and Kirstin Mitchell, 2010.

10 Jim Pfaus, committee # 7 presentation at the ICSM 3 conference in Paris, 10–13 July 2009.

11 K. Park, I. Goldstein & C. Andry et. al., 'Vasculogenic female sexual dysfunction: The hemodynamic basis for vaginal engorgement insufficiency and clitoral erectile insufficiency', *International Journal of Impotence Research*, vol. 9, 1997, pp. 27–37.

12 L. Tiefer, 'The medicalisation of sexuality: Conceptual normative and professional issues', *Annual Review of Sex Research*, vol. 7, 1996, pp. 252–82.

13 R. Moynihan, 'The making of a disease: female sexual dysfunction', *BMJ*, vol. 326, 2003, pp. 45–7.

14 Lori Brotto, committee # 24 presentation at the ICSM 3 conference in Paris, 10–13 July 2009.

15 A. Kinsey et. al., *Sexual Behavior in the Human Female*, W.B. Saunders, New York, 1953, p. 594.

16 ibid., p. 721.

17 Goldstein et. al., *Women's Sexual Function and Dysfunction*, Ch. 10.2. The quoted word 'normal' in the previous line comes from this chapter.

18 Annamaria Giraldi, committee # 22 presentation at the ICSM conference in Paris, 10–13 July 2009.

19 P. Abramson, 'Sexual science: Emerging discipline or oxymorons', *Journal of Sex Research*, vol. 27, 1990, p. 153.

20 Ray Rosen committee # 6 presentation at the ICSM 3 conference in Paris, 10–13 July 2009.

21 R. Rosen, C. Brown, J. Heiman et. al., 'The Female Sexual Function Index (FSFI): A multidimensional self-report instrument for the assessment of Female Sexual Function', *Journal of Sex & Marital Therapy*, vol. 26, 2000, pp. 191–208.

22 Business Wire story, 'Clinical results from Zonagen's Vasofem study show promise for treatment of Female Sexual Dysfunction', Texas, 7 September 2000, http://findarticles.com/p/articles/mi_m0EIN/is_2000_Sept_7/ai_65062478/.

23 http://www.fsfi-questionnaire.com.

24 Goldstein et. al., *Women's Sexual Function and Dysfunction*, Ch. 11.2.

25 D. Shames, S. Monroe, D. Davis & L. Soule, 'Regulatory perspective on clinical trials and end points for female sexual dysfunction, in particular, hypoactive sexual desire disorder: Formulating recommendations in an environment of evolving clinical science', *International Journal of Impotence Research*, vol. 19, 2007, pp. 30–6.

26 Business Wire, 'Clinical results from Zonagen's Vasofem study'.

27 F. Quirk, J. Heiman & R. Rosen et. al., 'Development of a sexual function questionnaire for clinical trials of Female Sexual Dysfunction', *Journal of Women's Health and Gender-based medicine*, vol. 11, 2002, pp. 277–89.

28 L. Derogatis, J. Rust & S. Golombok et. al., 'Validation of the profile of Female Sexual Function (PFSF) in surgically and naturally menopausal women', *Journal of Sex & Marital Therapy*, vol. 30, 2004, pp. 25–36; C. McHorney, J. Rust & S. Golombok et. al., 'Profile of Female Sexual Function', *Menopause*, vol. 11, 2004 pp. 474–83.

29 Review by the Division of reproductive and Urologic Drug Products, 3 November 2004, Intrinsa, NDA 21–769, p. 25.

30 Kirstin Mitchell writes in her PhD thesis that biomedical aspects of function are assessed because a lot of questionnaires are specifically designed to provide concise end points in clinical trials. K. Mitchell, Sexual Dysfunction: Conceptual and Measurement Issues, unpublished doctoral dissertation, London School of Hygiene and Tropical Medicine, 2008.

31 Ray Rosen's committee # 6 presentation at ICSM 3 conference in Paris, 10–13 July 2009.

32 ibid.

33 Boehringer Ingelheim press release, 'New diagnostic tool helps health care professionals accurately diagnose Hypoactive Sexual Desire Disorder (HSDD) in women', 3 March 2009.

34 A. Clayton, E. Goldfischer & I. Goldstein et. al., 'Validation of the Decreased Sexual Desire Screener (DSDS): A brief diagnostic instrument for Generalised Acquired Female Hypoactive Sexual Desire Disorder (HSDD)', *Journal of Sexual Medicine*, published online 13 January 2009.

35 Boehringer press release, 'New research shows emotional impact of low sexual desire and associated distress', 18 February 2010, http://www.eurekalert.org/pub_releases/2010–02/opr-nrs021710.php.

36 A. Clayton et. al., 'Validation of the Decreased Sexual Desire Screener'.

37 Ray Moynihan interview with Lori Brotto, 2009.

Chapter 4   Educating doctors with ski trips and strip clubs

1 See The Mansion website www.mansиononturtlecreek.com.

2 See details of the settlement at www.stopmedicarefraud.gov/pfizerfactsheet. html.

3 'Settlement agreement', p. 6. Despite repeated invitations, Pfizer declined an interview for this book, to talk about the allegations related to the settlement among other matters.

4 J. Robertson & R. Moynihan et. al., 'Mandatory disclosure of pharmaceutical industry-funded events for health professionals', *PLoS Medicine*, vol. 6, 2009, epub, 3 November.

5 For the best collection of all the relevant studies, see www.healthyskecpticism.org.

6 Much of this early section of the chapter is based on the 194-page complaint filed by lawyers acting for Blair Collins, filed in August 2007. The document is titled, 'Civil Action No. 04-11780 DPW, Restated and Amended False Claims Act Complaint, United States District Court for the District of Massachusetts'.

7 S. Boseley, 'Drug firm censured for lapdancing junket', *The Guardian*, 14 February 2006.

8 See www.stopmedicarefraud.gov/pfizerfactsheet.html.

9 For more information, see the Pharmed Out site http://pharmedout.org. Also see the Consumers International campaign called 'Marketing Overdose', www.marketingoverdose.org, and associated videos at www.youtube. com/view_play_list?p=98D188FFB287A9E4.

10 This material with Kimberly Elliott comes from R. Moynihan, 'Key opinion leaders: Independent experts or drug representatives in disguise?', *BMJ*, vol. 336, 2008, pp. 1402–3.

11 ibid.

12 R. Moynihan, 'Doctors' education: The invisible influence', *BMJ*, vol. 336, 2008, pp. 416–17.

13 D. Rothman, Industry support and professional medical associations— reply (letter), *JAMA*, vol. 302, 2009, http://jama.ama-assn.org/cgi/ content/extract/302/7/739–b. Also see S. Fletcher, 'Continuing education in the health professions: Improving healthcare through lifelong learning. Chairman's summary of the conference', Josiah Macy Jr

Foundation, New York, 2008.

14 M. Steinman et. al., 'Narrative review: The promotion of gabapentin. An analysis of internal industry documents', *Annals of Internal Medicine*, vol. 145, 2006, pp. 284–93.

15 Fletcher, 'Continuing education in the health professions'.

16 R. Moynihan, 'The making of a disease: female sexual dysfunction', *BMJ*, vol. 326, 2003, pp. 45–7. Much of the material in this section comes from this journal article.

17 R. Moynihan, 'Urologist recommends daily Viagra to prevent impotence', *BMJ*, vol. 326, 2003, p. 9 . This section of the book draws from this news story in *BMJ*.

18 *Speakers guide, Sexual health hospital Symposia, half-day CME Program*, National Foundation for Sexual Health Medicine. The material in this section is drawn from this document.

19 See www.fsfiquestionnaire.com.

20 *Renewing Sexual Desire: Understanding HSDD in postmenopausal women*. Slides and materials pertaining to a presentation on 20 November 2004.

21 Personal communication with Leonore Tiefer.

22 www.femalesexualdysfunctiononline.org/site/editorial.cfm (site since closed).

23 See R. Moynihan, W. Carlisle & M. Burne, 'Paying the medical piper', ABC Radio National, *Background Briefing*, 24 February 2008, www.abc. net.au/rn/backgroundbriefing/stories/2008/2166307.htm; R. Moynihan, 'Doctors' education' and R. Moynihan, 'Health seminars spruik drug firms', *The Australian*, 22 February 2008.

24 S. Fletcher, 'Continuing education in the health professions'.

25 Faculty and speaker disclosure, ISSWSH Annual Meeting, 28–31 October 2004, Atlanta.

26 International Society for the Study of Women's Sexual Health, ISSWSH Annual Meeting, 28–31 October 2004, Atlanta, conference book includes abstracts.

27 R. Moynihan, 'Key opinion leaders: independent experts or drug representatives in disguise?', *BMJ*, vol. 336, 2008, pp. 1402–3.

28 Pfizer response to Ray Moynihan's questions, 2010.

29 http://jsm.issir.org/ (accessed 7 April 2009).

30 S. Goldstein, 'My turn . . . finally' (editorial), *Journal of Sexual Medicine*, vol. 6, 2009, pp. 301–2.

31 K. Zucker & J. Cantor, 'The archives in the era of online first ahead of print', *Archives of Sexual Behavior*, vol. 37, 2008, pp. 512–16.

32 J. Pfaus, 'Aberrational Blots or Practice Shots? The Impact of "Self-Citation"' (editorial), *Journal of Sexual Medicine*, vol. 6, 2009, pp. 897–8.

33 Ray Moynihan interview with John Dean, 2009.

34 L. Tiefer, 'Beneath the veneer: The troubled past and future of sexual medicine', *Journal of Sex & Marital Therapy*, vol. 33, 2007, pp. 473–7.

35 Pfizer Fact Sheet, on a site called Stop Medicare Fraud, jointly hosted by the US Department of Health and Human Services and Justice, www.stopmedicarefraud.gov/pfizerfactsheet.html.

36 Sentencing hearing, Justice Douglas Woodlock, District Court of Massachusetts, 16 October 2009, p. 6–8.

37 J. Edwards, 'Pfizer rep claims Zoloft touted for failed cheerleaders', Viagra for Women, *Bnet*, 9 September 2009, http://industry.bnet.com/pharma/10004174/pfizer-rep-claims-zoloft-touted-for-failed-cheerleaders-viagra-for-women.

Chapter 5   Viagra turns twelve

1 P. Conrad & V. Leiter, 'From Lydia Pinkham to Queen Levitra: direct-to-consumer advertising and medicalistation', *Sociology of Health & Illness*, vol. 30, 2008, pp. 825–38.

2 H. Feldman, I. Goldstein, D. Hatzichristou, R. Krane & J. McKinlay, 'Impotence and its medical and psychological correlates: Results of the Massachusetts Male Aging Study', *Journal of Urology*, 151, 1994, pp. 54–61. Also see D. Tuller, 'Sex and medicine: Gentlemen start your engines', *The New York Times*, 21 June 2004, www.nytimes.com/2004/06/21/health/sex-medicine-gentlemen-start-your-engines.html?pagewanted=1.

3 J. Lexchin, 'Bigger and better: How Pfizer redefined erectile dysfunction', *PLoS Medicine*, vol. 3, 2006, e132. doi:10.1371/journal.pmed.0030132.

4 ibid.

5 The ad featured in the March 2002 issue of *Popular Science*.

6 US Congressional Budget Office, *Promotional Spending for Prescription Drugs*, economic and budget issue brief, 2 December 2009.

7 M. Gagnon & J. Lexchin, 'The cost of pushing pills: A new estimate of pharmaceutical promotion expenditures in the United States', *PLoS Medicine*, vol. 5, 2008, e1. doi:10.1371/journal.pmed.0050001.

8 J. Baglia, *The Viagra (Ad) Venture*, Peter Lang, New York, 2005, p. 72. Cited from R. Watson, 'The globe is gaga for Viagra', *Newsweek*, 22 June 1998, p. 44. Also see www.dreamcream.com.au/team/Kaminetsky.asp.

9 J. Simons, 'Taking on Viagra . . .', *Fortune Magazine*, vol. 147, 2003, pp. 102–12.

10 Pfizer advertisement in *The Weekend Australian*, 2/3 March 2002, p. 5.

11 The advertisement came from *The Good Weekend*, 2000.

12 The advertisement referenced an abstract, later published in full as K. Chew et. al., 'Erectile dysfunction in general medicine practice: Prevalence and clinical correlates', *International Journal of Impotence Research*, vol. 12, 2000, pp. 41–5.

13 U. Malmsten, I. Milsom, U. Molander & L. Norlen, 'Urinary incontinence and lower urinary tract symptoms: an epidemiological study of men aged 45 to 99 years', *Journal of Urology*, vol. 158, 1997, pp. 1733–7.

14 I. Spector & M. Carey, 'Incidence and prevalence of the sexual dysfunctions: A critical review of the empirical literature', *Archives of Sexual Behavior*, vol. 19, 1990, pp. 389–408.

15 H. Feldman et. al., 'Impotence and its medical and psychological correlates.

16 Lexchin, 'Bigger and better'.

17 K. Kleinman, H. Feldman & C. Johannes, 'A new surrogate variable for erectile dysfunction status in the Massachusetts male aging study', *Journal of Clinical Epidemiology*, vol. 53, 2000, pp. 71–8.

18 www.sortedin10.co.uk/erectile-dysfunction/understanding-ed.htm.

19 K. Waack, M. Ernst & M. Graber, 'Informational content of official pharmaceutical industry web sites about treatments for erectile dysfunctions', *Annals of Pharmacotherapy*, vol. 38, 2004, pp. 2029–34.

20 www.40over40.ca.

21 World Health Organization, *Ethical Criteria for Medicinal Drug Promotion*, WHO, Geneva, 1988.

22 Lilly response to Ray Moynihan, 2010.

23 C. Asberg & E. Johnson, 'Viagra selfhood: Pharmaceutical advertising and the visual formation of Swedish masculinity', *Health Care Anal*, vol. 17, 2009, pp. 144–57.

24 E. Johnson, 'Chemistries of love: Impotence, erectile dysfunction and Viagra in Lakartidningen', *Nordic Journal for Masculinity Studies*, vol. 3, 2008, pp. 31–47.

25 B. Mintzes, *Blurring the Boundaries: New Trends in Drug Promotion*, HAI-Europe Amsterdam, 1998. Available at www.haiweb.org; J. Lexchin, 'Bigger and better'.

26 H. Hedelin & L. Jacobsson, 'Viagra forstahandsmedel mor erektil dysfunction', *Lakartidningen*, vol. 97, 2000, pp. 2616–17. (Translated text and interpretation, E. Johnson, 'Chemistries of love: Impotence, erectile dysfunction and Viagra in Lakartidningen', *Nordic Journal for Masculinity Studies*, vol. 3, 2008, pp. 31–47.)

27 L. Tiefer, 'The Viagra Phenomenon', *Sexualities*, vol. 9, 2006, pp. 273–94; also Ray Moynihan interview with Leonore Tiefer, 2010.

28 A. Burls, W. Clark, L. Gold & S. Simpson, 'Sildenafil—an oral drug for the treatment of male erectile dysfunction', Birmingham (United Kingdom):

West Midlands Health Technology Assessment Collaboration, Department of Public Health and Epidemiology, University of Birmingham, 1998 Report number 12, www.rep.bham.ac.uk/1998/sildenafil.pdf.

29   M. Vardi & A. Nini, 'Phosphodiesterase inhibitors for erectile dysfunction in patients with diabetes mellitus', *Cochrane Database of Systematic Reviews*, vol. 1, 2007, CD002187. DOI: 10.1002/14651858.CD002187.pub3.

30   C. Miles, B. Candy & L. Jones et. al., 'Interventions for sexual dysfunction following treatments for cancer', *Cochrane Database of Systematic Reviews*, vol. 4, 2007, CD005540. DOI: 10.1002/14651858.CD00540.pub.2.

31   A. Tsertsvadze, F. Yazdi & H.A. Fink et. al., 'Oral sildenafil citrate (Viagra) for erectile dysfunction: A systematic review and meta-analysis of harms', *Urology*, vol. 74, 2009, pp. 831–6.

32   US Food and Drug Administration, Sildenafil Citrate (marketed as Viagra) Information, November 2007, www.fda.gov/Drugs/DrugsSafety/PostmarketDrugSafetyInformationforPatientsandProviders/ucm162833.htm.

33   T. Melnik, B. Soares & A. Nasello, 'Psychosocial interventions for erectile dysfunction', *Cochrane Database of Systematic Reviews*, vol. 3, 2007, CD004825. DOI: 10.1002/14651848.CD004825.pub2.

34   S. Linnebur, 'Tobacco education: Emphasising impotence as a consequence of smoking', *Am J Health-Syst Pharm*, vol. 63, 2006, pp. 2509–12; K. Park, J. Ku, S. Kim & J. Paick, 'Risk factors in predicting a poor response to sildenafil citrate in elderly men with erectile dysfunction', *BJU International*, vol. 95, 2005, pp. 366–70.

35   P.C. Souverein et. al., 'Incidence and determinants of sildenafil (dis)continuation in a Dutch cohort of sildenafil users', *International Journal of Impotence Research*, vol. 14, 2002, pp. 259–65; Y. Sato et. al., 'How long do patients with erectile dysfunction continue to use sildenafil citrate? Dropout rate from treatment course as outcome in real life', *International Journal of Urology*, vol. 14, 2007, pp. 339–42.

36   *AARP The Magazine*, 'Sexuality at midlife and beyond', 2004, update of attitudes and behaviors, conducted by TNS NFO Atlanta, Washington DC, May 2005.

37   S. Jacoby, 'Sex in America', *AARP Magazine*, July 2005, www.aarpmagazine.org/lifestyle/relationships/sex_in_america.html.

38   A. Potts, N. Gavey, V. Grace & T. Vares, 'The downside of Viagra: Women's experiences and concerns', *Sociology of Health & Illness*, vol. 25, 2003, pp. 697–719.

39   M. Loe, *The Rise of Viagra*, New York University Press, New York, 2004.

40   Lexchin, 'Bigger and better'.

41 T. Delate, V. Simmons & B. Motheral, 'Patterns of use of sildenafil among commercially insured adults in the United States: 1998–2002', *International Journal of Impotence Research*, vol. 16, 2004, pp. 313–18.

42 S.A.W. Shakir et. al., 'Cardiovascular events in users of sildenafil: Results from first phase of prescription event monitoring in England', *BMJ*, vol. 322, 2001, pp. 651–2; N. Dunn, 'Paper does not provide any reassurances', *BMJ*, vol. 323, 2001, p. 50.

43 C. Smith, Division of Drug Marketing, Advertising and Communication, US FDA, Letter to Robert Clark, Vice President, US Regulatory, Pfizer Inc. Re NDA # 20–895. Viagra (sildenafil citrate) tablets. MACMIS ID # 12726. Rockvile MD: 11/10/04.

44 J. Warren, 'In an oversexed age, more guys take a pill', *New York Times*, 14 December 2003.

45 J. Paul, et al., 'Viagra (sildenafil) use in a population-based sample of U.S. men who have sex with men', *Sexually Transmitted Diseases*, vol. 32, 2005, pp. 531–3.

46 L. Richwine, 'AIDS group sues Pfizer over Viagra ads', 22 January 2007, Reuters, Washington, DC, www.reuters.com/article/idUSN1736907320070122. AIDS group sues Pfizer over Viagra ads for "off-label" use', *AIDS Policy & Law*, vol. 22, 2007.

47 'Resisting prescribing pressure for sildenafil', *The Lancet*, vol. 369, 2007, p. 344.

48 J. Baglia, *The Viagra (Ad) Venture*.

Chapter 6 Premature prescriptions

1 Coverage of the meeting, including the incident on p. 157, is based on Ray Moynihan's notes from the day. Also L. Tiefer, 'Showdown in Gaithersburg: The New View report on the FDA Advisory Committee hearing on Procter & Gamble's testosterone patch, "Intrinsa"', 2 December 2004.

2 The material in this paragraph comes from R. Moynihan, 'Fix for low sex drive puts reporters in a bad patch', *BMJ*, vol. 329, 2004, p. 1294.

3 Press release, 'Landmark clinical study shows testosterone patch significantly improved sexual desire in surgically menopausal women', 4 May 2004.

4 R. Moynihan, 'The marketing of a disease: Female sexual dysfunction', *BMJ*, vol. 330, 2005, pp. 192–4. The quote from P&G comes from this paper as well.

5 Writing Group for the Women's Health Initiative Investigators, 'Risks and benefits of estrogen plus progestin in healthy postmenopausal women', *JAMA*, vol. 288, 2002, pp. 321–33.

6   S. Vedantam, 'FDA urged withholding data on antidepressants', *The Washington Post*, 10 September 2004.

7   Merck press release, Merck Announces Voluntary Worldwide Withdrawal of VIOXX®, 30 September 2004, www.merck.com/newsroom/vioxx/pdf/vioxx_press_release_final.pdf.

8   J. Berman, L. Berman & H. Lin et. al., 'Effect of sildenafil on subjective and physiologic parameters of the female sexual response in women with sexual arousal disorder', *Journal of Sex & Marital Therapy*, vol. 27, 2001, pp. 411–20.

9   R. Basson, R McInnes & M. Smith et. al., 'Efficacy and safety of sildenafil citrate in women with sexual dysfunction associated with female sexual arousal disorder', *Journal of Women's Health and Gender-based Medicine*, vol. 11, 2002, pp. X.

10 G. Harris, 'Pfizer gives up testing Viagra on women', *New York Times*, 28 February 2004.

11 All quotes are from Ray Moynihan's notes. Also see Moynihan, 'The marketing of a disease: female sexual dysfunction'.

12 See Review by the Division of Reproductive and Urologic Drug Products, 3 November 2004, Intrinsa, NDA 21–769, p. 25.

13 www.emea.europa.eu/humandocs/PDFs/EPAR/intrinsa/063406en6.pdf.

14 D. Martin, 'The female Viagra hits the NHS', *The Daily Mail,* 27 March 2007, www.dailymail.co.uk/health/article-444518/The-female-Viagra-hits-NHS.html.

15 MTRAC review: Inadequate evidence to support prescribing of testosterone patch (Intrinsa), Midlands Therapeutics Review and Advisory Committee, 15 November 2007, www.nelm.nhs.uk/en/NeLM-Area/News/492550/492714/492724.

16 'Testosterone patches for female sexual dysfunction', *Drugs and Therapeutics Bulletin*, vol. 47, 2009, pp. 30–4.

17 'Patch to perk up women's libido has little effect', *The Daily Mail*, 3 March 2009, www.dailymail.co.uk/health/article-1158722/Patch-perk-womens-libido-little-effect.html.

18 'Testostérone en patch (Intrinsa): Pas pour stimuler le désir feminine', *La Revue Prescrire*, vol. 27, 2007, p. 409.

19 L. Johnson, 'Warner Chilcottt buys P&G drug division', *Drug Discovery and Development*, 26 August 2009, www.dddmag.com/news-Warner-Chilcott-Buys-PG-Drug-Division-082509.aspx. See also Nasdaq, company news, 'Warner Chilcott agrees to acquire prescription-drug business of P&G for $3.1 bln cash—update', www.nasdaq.com/aspx/company-news-story.aspx?storyid=200908241033rttraderusequity_0652.

20   A. Bradford & C. Meston, 'Placebo response in the treatment of women's sexual dysfunctions: A review and commentary', *Journal of Sex & Marital Therapy*, vol. 35, 2009, pp. 164–81.

21   Ray Moynihan's interviews with Cindy Meston, 2009, 2010.

22   G. Braunstein, D. Sundwall & M. Katz et. al., 'Safety and efficacy of a testosterone patch for the treatment of hypoactive sexual desire disorder in surgically menopausal women, a randomised, placebo-controlled trial', *Archives of Internal Medicine*, vol. 165, 2005, pp. 1582–9, http://archinte.ama-assn.org/cgi/content/full/165/14/1582.

23   'Testosterone patches for female sexual dysfunction', *Drugs and Therapeutics Bulletin*, vol. 47, 2009, pp. 30–4.

24   C. Meston, 'The placebo response in women's sexuality research', State of The Art Lecture to the Annual Meeting of the International Society for the Study of Women's Sexual Health (ISSWSH), Florence, Italy, February 2009.

25   Third International Conference on Sexual Medicine, ICSM conference, Paris, 10–13 July 2004.

26   A. Clayton, E. Goldfischer & I. Goldstein et. al., 'Validation of the decreased sexual desire screener (DSDS): A brief diagnostic instrument for generalised acquired female hypoactive sexual desire disorder (HSDD)', *Journal of Sexual Medicine*, published online 13 January 2009; reprinted article distributed at the ICSM 3 conference, 10–13 July, Paris, 2009.

27   Ray Moynihan's notes from ICSM 3 conference.

28   D. Shames, S. Monroe, D. Davis & L. Soule, 'Regulatory perspective on clinical trials and end points for female sexual dysfunction, in particular, hypoactive sexual desire disorder: Formulating recommendations in an environment of evolving clinical science', *International Journal of Impotence Research*, vol. 19, 2007, pp. 30–6.

29   For a good discussion of conflict of interest, see S. Lewis, 'Neoliberalism, conflict of interest, and the governance of health research in Canada', *Open Medicine.* vol. 4, 2010, www.openmedicine.ca/article/view/379/302.

30   See symbol at www.ama-assn.org.

31   See the website at www.neriscience.com/web/default.asp.

32   See R. Rosen, J. Brewer & E. Gerstenberger et. al., 'Validation of the FSFI sexual desire domain diagnostic cut-point in predicting HSDD: Independent replication and confirmation', Abstract, at ICSM 3, 10–13 July 2009, Paris, http://icsm2009.meetingsevents.org/website/uploads/files/34%20Rosen.pdf.

33   D. Shames, S. Monroe, D. Davis & L. Soule, 'Regulatory perspective on clinical trials and end points for female sexual dysfunction, in particular, hypoactive sexual desire disorder: formulating recommendations in

an environment of evolving clinical science', *International Journal of Impotence Research*, vol. 19, 2007, pp. 30–6.

34 I. Goldstein, C. Meston, S. Davis & A. Traish (eds), *Women's Sexual Function and Dysfunction*, Taylor & Francis, Boca Raton, 2006, Chs 6.4, 11.3, 11.4 & 12.1.

Chapter 7 Undoing the disorders

1 Ray Moynihan interviews with Petra Boynton, 2009, 2010.

2 See www.halpern.co.uk.

3 'Searching for Sappho—exploring the legacy of the famous ancient Greek poet', ABC Radio, *Poetica* program, 10 October 2009, www.abc.net.au/rn/poetica/stories/2009/2664694.htm; Madonna, 'Burning Up'.

4 Boehringer press release, 'Women suffering from decreased sexual desire: Silence hinders diagnosis of the prevalent condition Hypoactive Sexual Desire Disorder (HSDD)', 7 May 2008.

5 Boehringer press release, 'New diagnostic tool helps health care professionals accurately diagnose Hypoactive Sexual Desire Disorder (HSDD) in women', 3 March 2009 uses the one-in-ten figure and quotes J. Shifren, B. Monz, P. Russo, A. Segreti & C. Johannes, 'Sexual problems and distress in United States women: Prevalence and correlates', *Obstetrics and Gynecology*, vol. 112, 2008, pp. 970–8.

6 R. Segraves & T. Woodard, 'Female hypoactive sexual desire disorder: History and current status', *Journal of Sexual Medicine*, vol. 3, 2006, pp. 408–18. This segment has relied on this history.

7 R. Balon & R. Segraves, *Handbook of Sexual Dysfunction*, Ch. 3 by Rosemary Basson.

8 See Boehringer press release, 'Women suffering from decreased sexual desire'. This press release states that: 'Research is ongoing to provide additional insight into flibanserin's specific mechanism of action.' Another document from the company, titled 'Flibanserin Background Information', dated November 2009, talks about the company's 'current understanding' and its beliefs in relation to how the drug might work.

9 See comments at http://biopsychiatry.com/misc/flibanserin.html.

10 Ray Moynihan interview with Leonore Tiefer, 2009.

11 B. Touhcet, J. Warnock, W. Yates & K. Wilkins, 'Evaluating the quality of websites offering information on female hypoactive sexual desire disorder', *Journal of Sex & Marital Therapy*, vol. 33, 2007, pp. 329–42.

12 Boehringer press release, 'Women suffering from decreased sexual desire.

13 Ray Moynihan interview with Petra Boynton, 2009.

14 HSDD Forum Programme, Hilton Hotel, London Tower Bridge, 17–18 September 2008.

15 See http://www.wizzard.co.uk.

16 Ray Moynihan interview with John Dean, 2009.

17 I. Goldstein, C. Lines, R. Pyke & J. Sheld, 'National Differences in patient-clinician communication regarding hypoactive sexual desire disorder', *Journal of Sexual Medicine*, vol. 6, 2009, pp. 1349–57.

18 The paper suggested feelings conveyed by patients included frustration, confusion, dissatisfaction and discontent, rather than distress.

19 Boehringer letter to Petra Boynton, 1 December 2009, www.drpetra.co.uk.

20 K. Klausner, 'Wyeth ghostwriting documents added to drug industry document archive', *PLoS Medicine* community blog, 18 September 2009, http://speakingofmedicine.plos.org/2009/09/18/wyeth-ghostwriting-documents-added-to-drug-industry-document-archive.

21 Drug industry document archive site, http://dida.library.ucsf.edu/pdf/rgc37b10.

22 R. Segraves & T. Woodard, 'Female hypoactive sexual desire disorder: History and current status', *Journal of Sexual Medicine*, vol. 3, 2006, pp. 408–18. This segment has relied on this history.

23 W. Masters & V. Johnson, *Human Sexual Inadequacy*, Little, Brown and Co., Boston, 1970, Ch. 13.

24 W. Masters, V. Johnson & R. Kolodny, *On Sex and Human Living*, Macmillan, London, 1982, p. 482.

25 L. Brotto, 'The DSM diagnostic criteria for hypoactive sexual desire disorder in women', *Archives of Sexual Behavior*, 24 September 2009, epub ahead of print.

26 ibid. and see C. Graham, 'The DSM diagnostic criteria for female sexual arousal disorder', *Archives of Sexual Behaviour*, 24 September 2009, epub ahead of print.

27 This is Kinsey being quoted in P. Robinson, *The Modernisation of Sex*, Harper and Row, New York, 1976, p. 111.

28 K. Garde & I. Lunde, 'Female sexual behavior: A study in a random sample of 40 year old women', *Maturitas*, vol. 2, 1980, pp. 225–40.

29 E. Laan & S. Both, 'What makes women experience desire?', *Feminism & Psychology*, vol. 18, 2008, pp. 505–14. This section is based on this paper and on Ray Moynihan's interview with Ellen Laan, 2009.

30 Ray Moynihan interview with Ellen Laan, 2009.

31 R. Balon & R. Segraves (eds), *Handbook of Sexual Dysfunction*, Ch. 3 by Rosemary Basson.

32 Brotto, 'The DSM diagnostic criteria for hypoactive sexual desire disorder in women'.

33 R. Basson, J. Berman & A. Burnett et. al., 'Report of the international

consensus development conference on female sexual dysfunction: Definitions and classifications', *Journal of Urology*, vol. 163, 2000, pp. 888–93.

34 ibid., p. 890. Also see the chapter by S. Leiblum, in I. Goldstein, C. Meston, S. Davis & A. Traish, *Women's Sexual Function and Dysfunction*, Taylor & Francis, Boca Raton, 2006, Ch. 9.1, p. 325.

35 R. Basson, S. Leiblum, L. Brotto, L. Derogatis, J. Fourcroy & K. Fugl-Meyer et. al., 'Definitions of women's sexual dysfunction reconsidered: Advocating expansion and revision', *Journal of Psychosomatic Obstetrics and Gynaecology*, vol. 24, 2003, pp. 221–9.

36 ibid.

37 C. Mercer, K. Fenton & A. Johnson et. al., 'Sexual function problems and help seeking behaviour in Britain: National probability sample survey', *BMJ*, vol. 327, 2007, pp. 426–7.

38 I. Nazareth, P. Boynton & M. King, 'Problems in sexual function with people attending London general practitioners: A cross sextional study', *BMJ*, vol. 327, 2003, p. 423.

39 See www.psych.org/MainMenu/Research/DSMIV/DSMV/BOTPrinciples.aspx.

40 Brotto, 'The DSM diagnostic criteria for hypoactive sexual desire disorder in women'.

41 Ray Moynihan interview with Leonore Tiefer, 2010.

42 Esquire website, 2005.

43 Ray Moynihan interview with Lori Brotto, 2009.

44 Materials sent to Ray Moynihan from Boehringer Ingelheim. The combined Europe and United States figures come from Abstract #008 from the Congress of the European Society for Sexual Medicine, E. Jolly et. al., 'Efficacy of flibanserin 100 mg qhs as a potential treatment for Hypoactive Sexual Desire Disorder in premenopausal women', 15–18 November 2009, Lyon.

45 http://www.fda.gov/downloads/AdvisoryCommittees/Committees MeetingMaterials/Drugs/ReproductiveHealthDrugsAdvisoryCommittee/UCM215437.pdf.

46 E. Laan & S. Both, 'What makes women experience desire?', *Feminism & Psychology*, vol. 18, 2008, pp. 505–14.

Chapter 8 Looking ahead

1 S. de Beauvoir, *The Second Sex*, Jonathan Cape, London, 1953, p. 686.

2 A. Ramachandran, 'Sexual dysfunction spray gets up experts' noses', *WAToday*, 24 April 2009, www.watoday.com.au/national/sexual-

dysfunction-spray-gets-up-experts-noses-20090424–ahn7.html.

3   See http://www.amiaustralia.com.au/female-sexual-dysfunction.

4   See http://www.sandiegosexualmedicine.com.

5   See http://www.wasvisual.com/lecture.html?lecture=322.

6   R. Rosen & G. Bachman, 'Sexual well-being, happiness and satisfaction in women: The case for a new conceptual paradigm', *Journal of Sex & Marital Therapy*, vol. 34, 2008, pp. 291–7.

7   J. Lexchin, L. Bero, B. Djulbegovic & O. Clark, 'Pharmaceutical industry sponsorship and research outcome and quality: Systematic review', *BMJ*, vol. 326, 2003, pp. 1167–70.

8   R. Moynihan, 'Doctors' education: The invisible influence', *BMJ*, vol. 336, 2008, pp. 416–17; S. Fletcher, 'Continuing education in the health professions: Improving healthcare through lifelong learning. Chairman's summary of the conference', Josiah Macy Jr Foundation, 2008, www.josiahmacyfoundation.org/documents/Macy_ContEd_I_7_08.pdfS.

9   A. Wazana, 'Physicians and the pharmaceutical industry: Is a gift ever just a gift?', *JAMA*, vol. 283, 2000, pp. 373–80.

10 See www.fsd-alert.org, www.nofreelunch.org, www.healthyskecticism.org.

11 Institute of Medicine report, 2009, *Conflict of Interest in Medical Research, Education, and Practice*, www.iom.edu/Reports/2009/Conflict-of-Interest-in-Medical-Research-Education-and-Practice.aspx.

12 S. Fletcher, 'Continuing education in the health professions'.

13 D. Rothman, W. MacDonald, C. Berkowitz & S. Shimonas et. al., 'Professional medical associations and their relationships with industry: A proposal for controlling conflict of interest', *JAMA*, vol. 301, 2009, pp. 1367–72, abstract at http://jama.ama-assn.org/cgi/content/abstract/301/13/1367.

14 F. Godlee, 'Doctors, patients, and the drug industry', *BMJ*, vol. 338, 2009, p. 463.

15 F. Godlee, 'Key opinion leaders your time is up', *BMJ*, vol. 336, 2008, p. 413.

16 See the press release at the time of the launch of the Act: http://aging.senate.gov/record.cfm?id=307097. For committee material on proposed laws see http://finance.senate.gov/sitepages/leg/LEG%202009/042809%20Health%20Care%20Description%20of%20Policy%20Option.pdf.

17 R. Moynihan & M. Sweet, *Ten Questions You Must Ask Your Doctor*, Allen & Unwin, Sydney, 2008.

18 B. Arndt, *The Sex Diaries*, Melbourne University Press, Melbourne, 2009, p. 81.

19 J. Sauers, *Sex Lives of Australian Women*, Random House, Sydney, 2008.

20 de Beauvoir, *The Second Sex*.

Index

RAY MOYNIHAN has been investigating the business of health care as a journalist for over a decade. He is the author and co-author of three previous books, including *Selling Sickness*, which has been translated into a dozen languages. He lives in Byron Bay, Australia.

DR. BARBARA MINTZES investigates the link between clinical trials and pharmacosurveillance evidence on drug safety and effectiveness. She is an Assistant Professor in the Department of Pharmacology & Therapeutics at the University of British Columbia.